Practical Budget Management in Health and Social Care

William Bryans

Unive
Subject

http

Radcliffe Publishing
Oxford • New York

Radcliffe Publishing Ltd
18 Marcham Road
Abingdon
Oxon OX14 1AA
United Kingdom

www.radcliffe-oxford.com
Electronic catalogue and worldwide online ordering facility.

British Library Cataloguing in Publication Data

A catalogue record for this book is available from the British Library.

ISBN-13: 978 184619 100 8

Typeset by Lapiz Digital Services, Chennai
Printed and bound by TJI Digital, Padstow, Cornwall

Contents

Preface

This book is the third in a series of three. They all share the same under-pinning philosophy. Regardless of changes to structure, organisation or methods of finance, the fundamental principles of good stewardship and financial rectitude are crucial to commissioning and delivering an effective and efficient service. Inherent are a number of critical factors:

- *Everyone* is involved in resource consumption. From the flick of a light switch to the use of the most advanced equipment and techniques, staff, patients, clients, relatives, members of the public, all spend the organisation's money. This means that financial and business management must have a wide spectrum of development features that seek to be inclusive.
- *Resources age.* Resources, including staff and possibly organisations, become old, obsolete or are overtaken by some new development, and need to be refreshed and replenished. Managers must ensure that they have the necessary systems and skills to promote their departments and keep them up-to-date.
- *Workloads are directly related to available resources.* However, for a wide variety of reasons, that relationship will differ from unit to unit. For example, because of lack of economies of scale in a smaller unit that has a lower workload, resource consumption will be higher on average. It follows that comparisons between units will therefore be difficult to make, with smaller units often at an immediate disadvantage.
- *There is no substitute for walking the floor.* Successful resource and budget managers have a reputation for close inspection of their territories. They try not to become too immersed in facts and figures but balance this activity by getting out of their offices into the workplace where they expect to find a busy but not impossible burden of work. There they are constantly listening, touching, smelling, seeing and making valuable external contacts. They take pride in a clean and tidy environment; are constantly seeking to improve staff morale by taking an interest in their problems. Effective managers practise process quality in financial and business management, and are alert to a range of both physical and intangible hazards. They want to make sure that their units are running properly. In the long run that is what keeps costs down.

There are therefore a range of structured activities that may be carried out independently of any budget report or spreadsheet: in due course they will become the core driving force that will keep costs down and budgets within limits. The logic of the three books follows these activities in a structured way so that managers can gradually implement a complete package:

- **Process quality in financial and business management:** This is the main theme of *Managing in Health and Social Care: essential checklists for frontline staff* and concentrates upon doing the right thing, first time, every time.
- **Matching available resources to the environment:** This is the main theme of *Resource Management in Health and Social Care: essential checklists* and deals with workplace and external environmental problems associated with resource scarcity.
- **Practical budget management** is at the core of this book. As well as giving an insight into the way budgets behave in certain circumstances and what can be done about it, the book also deals with practical steps the budget and resource manager can take to eliminate waste and reduce opportunities for fraud and collusion.

William Bryans
January 2007

About the author

William Bryans is a specialist in health and social care business and financial management. He has wide ranging senior management experience of resource management in Northern Ireland's integrated health and social care system including membership of Belfast's famous Royal Hospital Group management team during the height of the troubles.

He also has experience in the commissioning, provision and management of hospital, residential and community services to the elderly, mentally ill, people suffering from physical handicap, people with learning difficulties and child care.

As a promoter of the workplace as a management college, he has lectured widely on the subject including postgraduate courses in health and social care management at the University of Ulster. He is a Fellow of the Chartered Institute of Secretaries and Administrators (FCIS) and a Fellow of the Institute of Health Care Management (FHCM).

In addition to his many contributions to 'Health Management', which is the official publication of the Institute of Healthcare Management, William Bryans was a founder member of the Northern Ireland branch of the Institute and for a number of years was a member of the Institute's panel of examiners. He also acted as external assessor for the Institute's MESOL (Management Education System through Open Learning) project.

This book follows closely upon the success of two previously published by Radcliffe:

> *Managing in Health and Social Care: essential checklists for frontline staff* (2004)
> *Resource Management in Health and Social Care: essential checklists* (2005).

About this book

Although there may be constant change to organisation and structures, great improvements in care, treatment and technology and ever more sophisticated ways of funding health and social care, the actual act of spending money will always be the responsibility of budget managers who are in the front line.

Practical Budget Management identifies the day-to-day issues that affect managers in health and social services, and provides advice and a structured approach that facilitate both comprehension of the problem areas and possible solutions. Each chapter includes:

- a list of main issues
- examples and illustrations where appropriate
- hints and tips for managers wishing to improve competence
- copious practical steps for managers confronted with specific problems
- numerous illustrative case studies and worked examples
- key point summary at the end.

This book is the third in a series published by Radcliffe, which provides practical solutions to the complex problems of resource, financial and budget management in health and social care. The first two titles are *Managing in Health and Social Care: essential checklists for frontline staff* and *Resource Management in Health and Social Care: essential checklists.*

Who will benefit?

There is a continuing deficit in the literature pertaining to practical aspects of budget management particularly in the context of worked examples. This book will therefore be of benefit and of practical assistance to managers, tutors, students, board members and other health and social care professionals who have an interest in the basics of this subject.

As with the other two books, better budget management means that the organisation can concentrate greater resources on those pressure issues, such as waiting list reductions, that will greatly enhance patient and client care. There is also greater scope to improve overall quality from initiatives that come from within the organisation and these will have a direct effect on staff safety, security, morale and sense of well-being. Benefits will also accrue to relatives and visitors, who will experience better support and a prevalent sense of improved confidence.

Cost reductions, either through greater through-put or savings or both, increase performance and provide a more secure basis for better accountability.

Case studies

As well as illustrating various points, the case studies are also intended as talking points for students, who should be encouraged to discuss them. However, whilst the case studies are based on real situations, all details such as names are pure fiction. Any resemblance or similarity to persons or places is completely coincidental.

This book is dedicated to my wife, Edith, without whose support it would never have been written.

Chapter 1

The budget management context

The issues

- It is often claimed that budgets and the need to 'balance the books' are the prime concerns of management.
- And, in the sense that our services would fold if we ran out of money, financial concerns and constraints are important considerations.
- However it is the inextricable link with the expectation, scope, quality and intensity of patient/client care, together with the availability of other resources, which forms the central issues that generate the escalating demand upon limited financial resources.
- Scarcity of physical and human assets is affected by a complex number of political and economic factors.
- These, together with clinical and technical advances that heighten expectation, are major pressures upon the limited money that is made available.
- Often, these factors appear outside the influence of the individual budget manager.
- But this should not be an inhibiting factor to the implementation of good practice.
- Managers need to become familiar with the context so that they comprehend the outer parameters.

Introduction

When, despite considerable additions to an already enormous budget that accounts for around 21% of public expenditure, there is a perpetual funding crisis in health and social care, we do not need a financial wizard to tell us that something is wrong. However, as pointed out in *Resource Management*,[1] it is important to keep big numbers in perspective – big budgets can experience big variations.

Although this book, unlike its predecessors, is primarily concerned with the behaviour of expenditure trends and the control and management of spending within defined limits, it is impossible to ignore the fact that spending on health and social care is a response to patient/client demand. However, the interaction of managers at various levels in the organisations concerned creates a rate of resource consumption that should reflect the effectiveness of care and treatment.

This chapter looks at those elements that contrive to limit the effectiveness of budgetary management. Whilst there are many elements that seem to lie outside the budget manager's sphere of influence, there are an enormous number of steps that can be taken to cope with the pressures generated by expectation and resource management.[2]

Political and economic factors

In recent years, the plight of patients/clients pleading for care or treatment that is readily available elsewhere seems to fly in the face of those treasured core values, equity and equality. Naturally there is considerable public support for such individuals, especially when the treatment is for life-threatening conditions, and there is little sympathy for official arguments for refusing care or treatment that depend upon, for example, the incredibly high cost of the drug in question. But what ingredient puts the prices quoted for monthly/yearly dosages beyond that of a precious metal? Sometimes it is hard to believe that such prices have been subjected to the rigorous scrutiny and influence of the massive purchasing power of the service.

On the other hand, and often in order to reduce waiting lists, the purchase of some of that care and treatment from external sources appears inconsistent with the effectiveness of internal provision and is likely at some stage to precipitate either further crisis in funding or service instability. For, in a situation where there are limited physical resources in the form of skilled staff, it seems likely that there must be some erosion of available expertise from within the service in favour of the private provider, and short-termism would appear to prevail.

With increasing numbers of vulnerable people in the community, services are also under constant pressure to both cope with providing the care required and live within the budgets allocated. Social service budgets also have to be managed in a way that ensures greater independence for clients and, in the case of children in social service care, a movement away from residential accommodation and towards fostering and adoption.

As with the rest of society, there is naturally a greater emphasis on people's rights and strenuous efforts are made to encourage supported family life where this is deemed appropriate. Generally, as with hospital and other services, there is also an escalating expectation of improvement in service provision and, as we have all observed, very little consideration for hard pressed staff when, for example, child protection fails.

The examples described above are high-profile problems, readily given media coverage. Nevertheless there seems to be an inherent suspicion that, despite being remote from policy and negotiation, local managers are responsible and should be accountable for the difficulties – perhaps unfairly.

However, at local level, but directly arising from these political and economic factors, there are a number of funding issues that require explanation, especially the effects of:

- growth and change, and how they affect budget management

- inflation and the need to reflect adequate funding by accurate budget adjustment
- the interpretation of 'big number' variations, particularly overspendings.

Growth in a climate of change

Having emerged from a long period of near-zero growth, during which hospitals and other long-term facilities were closed and the contracting out of certain internal services was immutable policy, it is little wonder that the current service, despite the infusion of considerable additional funding, is still under pressure. In these circumstances it is hard not to see a connection between the overuse of resources and the increases in life-threatening conditions such as MRSA.

There can be little doubt therefore that whilst we must all have our eyes upon the cost and appropriateness of care, it is more important to ensure that other factors, especially those less obvious to the layman, are not ignored. It is only when the 'quality' issue is firmly under control and patients/clients are no longer at risk, that more radical resource management measures are possible.

In *Resource Management*,[3] I drew attention to the importance of matching the level of care provided to the cost of care in terms of the resources consumed. This is a goal that is commensurate with both the release of physical resources and the potential for better and speedier availability of care and treatment for those at various stages where patients and clients have to wait for the next stage in their care/treatment to commence. It also reflects the fashionable notion of always providing care and treatment at the most appropriate level of dependency, thus ensuring that resources are not wasted.

However once a patient/client is discharged from longer-term care and requires continuing support in the community, the cost benefits arising from care are debatable. Indeed it seems likely that the economies of scale derived from concentrating resources in places like hospitals are diminished when the balance is shifted in favour of the community. Although the care, treatment and maintenance of patients/clients in their own homes are worthy and desirable facets of the overall care continuum, this is nevertheless an area where efficiency and effectiveness may not always be compatible.

Major difficulties as far as care provision is concerned are the many problems connected with the achievement of a seamless service. For example, in *The Health and Social Care Divide*,[4] the authors relate research findings to coherent and so called 'seamless service' provision and draw attention to the confusion that sometimes arises from the lack of clear delineation of service boundaries and the reluctance to accept financial responsibilities. Detrimental effects on the care available to patients/clients, especially those with complex requirements, are inescapable. When it comes to the central issues of the efficacy of partnership, collaboration and cooperation at the interface, there is little disagreement amongst dedicated fieldworkers and front-line hospital staff, whose efforts to find appropriate levels of care for vulnerable patients/clients and carers can be so easily frustrated by organisational hazards, differing cultures, difficult moral and legal problems, complex administrative arrangements, etc. Amongst the recommendations in the Government's 10-year plan for the care of the elderly, the need for partner organisations to ensure continued joint working arrangements is highlighted.

Increasingly, the acute sector displays trends that suggest the desire to match appropriate dependency with resource implications. It is a characteristic of medical advances that sophisticated treatments such as dialysis are often undertaken under strict supervision in hospital, but as knowledge or further advances are made some patients can be cared for at home. And, in addition to the growth of day surgery and other day care treatments, conditions such as asthma and some heart problems, which were previously deemed to require hospital treatment, are considered suitable for care at home. However, the consequence of reducing hospital workloads in this way is that funding also ceases as a result of diminished commissioning. If the impact of this is severe, then a reduced budget will result in overspending, unless there is also a reduction in physical and human resources.

Balanced against this, there is a constant stream of approved new or improved services coming on-stream, which will attract appropriate additional funds.

Balance and quality of care

In order to make the best use of resources, and at the same time improve the quality of care, there has to be a great deal of emphasis upon finding the lowest appropriate level of care that is commensurate with patient/client requirements. Theoretically, through this process, scarce resources are released to meet other competing demands.

However this is in itself a complicated and difficult task, which has to embrace the constant increase in expectations from patients/clients/relatives/public and constant advances in scientific development.[5] These elements have in turn to be balanced against a consistent conservative reaction that inhibits progress, often with good reason.

Organisational and bureaucratic inhibitors

In complex organisations such as those devoted to health and social care, internal structures are created to reflect the diversity of specialisms within the organisational envelope. Each specialism, whether it is on the business side of the organisation or whether it is devoted to direct patient/client care, is dependent upon others so that together the whole should produce a comprehensively effective multidisciplinary approach to care and treatment.

To an extent these separate entities reflect the wide variety of patient/client requirements. However, the need to sustain professional integrity, develop skills and encourage innovation often leads to intro-verted attitudes that can be detrimental to the holistic approach. It can also mean that the movement or discharge of patients/clients to other parts of the organisation more appropriate to their needs becomes more difficult and the process, if there is one, more prolonged.

In a growing litigious climate, in which previously a less paper-oriented system may have prevailed and been acceptable, legal aspects now have to be carefully considered and proper documentation maintained. However, this growth in what appears to be unstoppable bureaucracy adds to the delays. Below are some of the better known examples.

- Protocols covering every aspect of patient/client care, which in extreme cases must include relatives' views and business aspects of the organisation, are increasingly necessary.
- When agreement between parties on ethical considerations has not been possible, for example, where there is a question of the continu-ation of life support, then distressingly these must be tested in court.
- When the relinquishing of independence or other life-changing decisions are necessary for the elderly or those with handicap, for example, after a stroke or an injury resulting in mobility problems, it is important to allow the patient/client/relative sufficient time and space in which to make informed choices.
- These delays may be alleviated by the efforts of a multidisciplinary care team.
- It is inevitable that these factors, together with the need to improve performance, will cause health and social care organisations to become risk averse.[6]
- In the hospital and residential sectors improvements in care, treatment, shifts in the balance of care and developments in technology increase the pressure to reduce beds and places, and further closures may be nec-essary in order to fund further developments. This gives rise to the need to give careful consideration to the consultative process.

Patient/client reactions

Patients/clients and their relatives do not always agree with the solutions to problems, including the current emphasis upon prevention rather than cure, that the professionals suggest. Frequently they are recalcitrant at accepting advice, attending clinics, or making life-changing decisions,

may be due in part to a lack of comprehension or a previous bad
ience. These elements also add complications to the time span
required to find the most appropriate level of care.

Where there is an unusual incidence of lack of agreement, it is worth
taking time to discover the cause. Here are a few examples (in addition to
those listed in *Resource Management*):[7]

- loss of confidence in advice that is open to challenge, for example,
  the efficacy of oily fish for heart problems or the promotion of
  healthy eating habits that may adversely affect certain conditions
- refusal of further medication that has already triggered violent
  symptoms of the disease
- refusal to attend unsolicited automatic appointments at nurse-led
  clinics
- reluctance on the part of the elderly and other vulnerable groups to
  reduce their independence.

Case study

Mr H O'Condriac, the chairman of the Bigtown patients' forum and hon-
orary governor of St Bedifuls Hospital, received a totally unexpected telephone call from St Bedifuls' day surgery unit, which, he was ashamed to
say, he had never visited. The caller informed him that a bed was available immediately for him to have a blood transfusion. As nobody had told
him his blood count was low or suggested that he might need a transfusion, his first reaction was one of shock, quickly followed by a feeling of
fear of blood transfusions. He therefore politely declined the transfusion
and determined to raise the matter at the next patients' forum meeting.

Resource implications

The thrust towards finding the level of care that is most appropriate to the
degree of patient/client dependency is well worthwhile in an integrated
health and social care system. However, where structures are not 'joined
up' it is debatable whether there are any financial benefits in this approach
because resources that were once concentrated would be more dispersed.

The basic reason for hospital and other residential provision has always
been based on the economies of scale arising from gathering high levels of
scarce expertise in one place. If we expect the same or similar levels of care
to be maintained in the community, then it is clear that costs and resource
consumption will rise significantly. If that situation cannot be sustained, it
follows that there have to be compromises in care at community level.

Resource consumption

Patient/client activity generates incredible demands for resources that are
on a constant upward trend. Increases in the total NHS budget have

prompted a growth from £34bn in 1997 to an estimated £92bn in 2006/7. According to the Health and Social Care Information Centre, expenditure on social services in England alone increased by 8% during 2005/6 to around £20bn. Although they are difficult to pin down, the main sources for these increases are:

- maintenance of standards in the face of escalating costs
- constant erosion of purchasing power through the debilitating effects of inflation which affects the costs of goods, services and personnel
- increases in the scope, range and diversity of services being offered (including controversial elements such as alternative therapies)
- general improvements in service provision through the availability of new monies to encourage growth in specifically designated areas, for example, increasing the number of doctors, nurses and social workers
- cost and impact of developments in IT, which are constantly in advance of strategic decisions
- replacing existing resources; in addition to the constant 'ordinary running cost' element and, more significantly, longer-term assets including staff that eventually require replacement.

Conclusion

Considering that the NHS on its own is credited with over 1.3m staff and social services with an estimated 0.4m at its disposal, it is clear that there is considerable scope for disjointed working. Indeed, on such a truly mammoth scale it seems inevitable that a whole spectrum of waste and inequalities would emerge and in many ways it is a commendable achievement that the system works so well.

Successful managers, in maintaining awareness of the areas where possible inefficiencies might arise and in recognising and taking opportunities to address and enhance the situation, clearly demonstrate that considerable savings can be made to the benefit of patients/clients.

Case study

Mr H O'Condriac received a long awaited appointment for the day surgery unit. Following several inquiries and blatantly using his status, Mr O'Condriac felt reassured that the delay was not due to the unpleasantness caused by his previous encounter with the unit management. He was to report for an examination at 7.45am.

Mr O'Condriac soon accumulated a list of complaints:

- he nearly missed the nondescript portacabin that housed the unit and he couldn't help but notice the rutted, overgrown car park
- on his way into the unit he noticed that the tiny seating area for relatives and carers was firmly locked, outside the main unit and had access to neither toilets nor beverages

- when he was taken to theatre, a nurse explained the procedure to him and pointed out a number of things that rarely went wrong
- the doctor asked him to remind him why he was having this particular procedure carried out
- when he arrived home, he tried to seek reassurance from his GP but wasn't quick enough to catch the answer-phone message beyond the fact that the after-hour arrangements had been changed.

In a way, Mr O'Condriac was pleased that he would have plenty of material for his opening remarks at the next patients' forum meeting.

Key point summary

- Budget managers are concerned to see that spending on resources and resource consumption are properly and efficiently applied to their workloads.
- In this capacity they are well used to coping with resource scarcities in available skills, space, materials, drugs, equipment, etc.
- Although budgets may be consistently overspent (difficult to reconcile with long lists of key staff vacancies), there are a number of factors that have to be considered.
- Levels of care appropriate to dependency will produce more efficient resource use.
- However excessive use of resources can be linked to negative influences on the quality of care.
- Movement of patients/clients out of a budget system, for example, from hospital to community care, results in loss of income to the hospital.

References

1 Bryans W. *Resource Management in Health and Social Care: essential checklists.* Oxford: Radcliffe Publishing; 2005. p. 80–81.
2 Ibid. p. 51–66.
3 Ibid. p. 63.
4 Glasby J, Littlechild R. *The Health and Social Care Divide: the experiences of older people.* Bristol: The Policy Press; 2004.
5 Bryans W. *Ibid.* Chapter 2.
6 Bryans W. *Ibid.* Chapter 4.
7 Bryans W. *Ibid.* Chapter 2.

External pressures and the efficacy of reporting an overspending

The issues

Despite the pessimism and budget managers' feelings of isolation from the upper levels where negotiation and other major policy decisions take place, there is however a great deal that they can do to improve their positions. This chapter examines various financial pressures that originate externally and the methods used to cope with them.

- Over time the insidious impact of inflationary pressure greatly reduces the purchasing power of budgets for goods, services and payroll.
- However, in addition to extra funding, there are a number of devices that can be employed to minimise the effects of inflation.
- Developments in technology, approved new services, improvements in service delivery such as increased staffing and building work may all be the subject of additional funding, although managers may have to bid for their share.
- If they are not already in the pipeline for additional funding, then managers must make sure that a suitable case is made.

Introduction

Budgets are under constant external pressure to cope with higher expectations and greater demands at minimal or no additional cost. These pressures are mainly manifested in the incidence of inflation, the constant need to keep up with improvements in new techniques and technology, changes in the way care and treatment are provided, and, as we have seen in Chapter 1, the development of new or improved services and staffing.

The insidious effects of inflation on budget management are apparent mainly in pay awards and price increases. Although various devices are used to reduce the impact, there are very few who enter a contract without some safeguard – even the *Titanic* was built on a cost-plus-percentage basis.

Pay awards

In the case of staff, it would be inconceivable that there should not be some consideration given to externally changing economic circumstances. It is also important to create stability in a highly skilled environment. Indeed, throughout the service it is the practice for staff to be paid according to a payscale as an acknowledgement of experience. As a result, where there is a low turnover and staff remain longer in post, the cost increases year by year through incremental drifting.

For many years there has also been official recognition of the extra expense incurred by those who work in the capital and especially for nursing staff as the availability of affordable accommodation has become more scarce. Variations in living costs across the regions have the potential to produce a greater staff supply where costs are lower and have a theoretical, if unpopular, potential for local pay arrangements that favour the organisation. Another implication, which may prove more fruitful in the long term, is the possibility of providing more cost effective back-office support from remote locations. This could be achieved through greater use of technology in the fields of records, finance and supplies, sourcing high quality staff in areas such as Northern Ireland where there is a surfeit.

Other increases in pay are sometimes awarded in productivity agreements or for the acceptance of improved staff structures. In theory such awards are inflation busting because they aim to produce better terms and conditions at the cost of a number of posts. However, their implementation is often difficult and may exceed whatever limit has been set in terms of cost.

Price increases

The detrimental effect of price increases is an unwanted phenomenon that hits everyone's pocket; health and social care provision suffers in much the same way through increased costs. All those items including drugs that are subject to price increases amount to around 20% of the day-to-day budget.

Because the various reference indices tend to be retrospective, it is much more difficult to measure the effects of price increases and make adjustments. Also, the basis of any given index can often be the cause of disagreement. This occurs where there is a perception that the 'shopping basket' that is used as a basis of measurement has some flaw. For example, if the price of oil, which in various forms is at the core of our economy, doubles in a year and massive profits are declared by the oil companies, yet there is no appreciable impact on the retail price index, then inevitably there would be some concern about the accuracy of the data.

Nevertheless, through the better use of market forces and massive purchasing power, it is possible to minimise the impact of increased costs. Within the supply chain, improvements in contract negotiation and vigilance in identifying competing suppliers who may form a collusive alliance to maintain higher prices result in better value for money.

Developments, improvements and new services

As well as the developments, improvements and new services for which budget managers have made formal bids,[1] there are others that subtly increase costs because of external market pressures and other influences.

Although these elements are fairly common throughout our services, they can be more prevalent on hospital, especially teaching hospital, sites where innovation, experiment, trials, etc. are important facets of a constantly evolving service.

In the case of smaller centres of activity and community services where there is constant pressure to develop new approaches to care and to promote partnerships with external organisations, many successful deals may be emerging that have cost consequences. Below is a short list of examples.

- **Purchasing and commissioning activities should be restricted to authorised and properly qualified staff**. One of the main contributory factors to uncontrolled spending is the reliance on non-purchasing staff to 'do a deal'.[2] This can even extend to unauthorised staff at ward or department level interviewing a trades representative and actually ordering an item or material. This is called vertical penetration and should be discouraged, except under certain controlled circumstances where a mutual exchange of views is necessary before committing to a particular purchase.
- **Topping up, planned preventative maintenance, and just-in-time (JIT)** arrangements are other possible areas for 'creeping growth'. Some form of spending control on these important techniques, such as bar coding, needs to be implemented if satisfactory budgetary management is to be achieved.
- **Short-term partnership contract reviews.** It is important to keep short-term contracts for staffing (for example, joint appointments with a university or other similar organisation and appointments where there is a financial contribution from another partner, such as in community care) under review. When the deadline is due to expire, terminate such appointments according to the rules and renew as appropriate.
- **Replacement upgrades.** When items and other resources become due for replacement (around five years in the case of electrical equipment), it is inevitable that managers may have to accept upgrades because of interim developments, as exemplified by the current pressure to change televisions and video recorders to digital technology. Managers may also be tempted to accept equipment that has unnecessary 'bells and whistles'. It can also happen that a new, upgraded item may have other cost implications such as an increased electricity or water usage, which will in turn have an unexpected impact on the budget.
- **Revenue consequences.** Often in addition to upgrades, capital expenditure attracts revenue consequences (running costs). This element may be
  — considered too insignificant to be included in calculations
  — a condition of accepting additional capital expenditure
  — overlooked altogether
  — underestimated and therefore underfunded.

Tips from the front office

- Review, terminate and renew short-term contracts, if this is appropriate.
- Assess the consequences of replacing furniture and equipment carefully.
- Make sure revenue consequences are always properly stated: underfunding will be a constant drain on scarce resources in the future.

Case study

Bigtown Hospital Trust has a total day-to-day budget of £100m. It has been estimated that over a year, a 3% price increase is required. This will add £600k to the goods and services budget. However, the newly appointed treasurer Midas Touchstone, reflecting current regional policy, feels that whilst there would be a 3% impact in a whole year, the increases came in gradually during the current year. In addition, the Trust has been participating, with some success, in a regional supply line initiative aimed at driving down prices by facilitating more competition and reducing cartels. Increases of this magnitude across the board are therefore believed to be unrealistic.

Reporting overspendings

Even in the best regulated situations, it seems inevitable that there would be some fluctuation about the budget target. It is only when overspendings appear to be out of control or there are no compensatory elements such as surpluses in other budgets that the situation becomes a matter for concern.

The context for this at any level of consolidation (national or local) is illustrated in Table 2.1, which shows a simple system of five budgets, A to E, with a reported spending S against a target T. By subtracting S from T the variation V is obtained and, depending on whether S exceeds T or T is the greater, the value of V will indicate an over- or underspending.

Table 2.1 Simplified budget overview

Budget	Target	Spend	Variation
A	T(a)	S(a)	V(a)
B	T(b)	S(b)	V(b)
C	T(c)	S(c)	V(c)
D	T(d)	S(d)	V(d)
E	T(e)	S(e)	V(e)
Totals	T(a+b+c+d+e)	S(a+b+c+d+e)	V(a+b+c+d+e)

Within a whole system, provided it was sufficiently large and there were no major underlying funding problems, there would usually be enough flexibility for the net position (V(a+b+c+d+e)) to be sustained by offsetting negative and positive variations against each other. But where all or most of the budgets were indicating major overspending then it seems likely that the difficulties would go further than normal housekeeping problems. Imagine that budget C has been set aside for a special project, which, although it was due to come on-stream from the beginning of the financial year, did not in fact become operational until half way through the year. All other things being equal, the variation V(c) will equal half the target, as shown in Table 2.2. This is an example of a windfall under-spending, which in that particular financial year will help compensate for overspendings elsewhere in the system.

Table 2.2   Underspending example

Budget	Target	Spending	Variation
C	T(c)	S(c)	V(c) = T/2

However, care should be taken the following year to take account of the full year's spending, which may in fact turn out to be at a higher level than the target T(c).

This demonstrates that if the actual cost of a resource or project turns out to be in excess of the finally agreed budget, it may be obscured, hidden or otherwise compensated for by the budget manager when all or some of the proposed purchase does not come on-stream in time.

Even so, it is important that we do not overlook the cumulative effects of underestimating an expected increase in the cost of new services or as the result of inflation. An underestimate in one year will be reflected in the following year, not just on a like-for-like basis, for the deficiency will be carried forward. Thus, an underestimate of £x in year 1 will become £10x in year 10. Furthermore if, in each successive year, a further deficit of £x occurred, by year 10 the total shortfall would be £55x. This is illustrated in Figure 2.1.

Case study

A few years ago in the Bigtown Hospital Trust a forecasted end-of-year overspending of £500k grabbed the headlines because it was offset by an almost identical underspending in the nearby Mental Health Trust and the media were fearful that this would signal a reallocation of resources. The fact that it represented only 0.5% of the total Bigtown Hospital Trust budget went unreported.

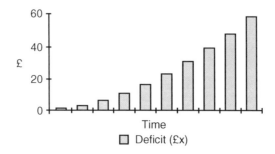

Figure 2.1 Cumulative deficits.

Tips from the front office

- In certain circumstances, health and social care providers can use overspendings as bargaining tools.
- However, commissioners will always be sceptical.

Key point summary

- An overspending may be due in part to underfunding of new services and inflation.
- And there are a number of other insidious pressures that may also be contributors.
- These aspects must be carefully monitored and action taken when appropriate.
- Overspending in one budget area can often be offset by an underspending in another.
- However this could produce concern that a reallocation of funds could disadvantage the latter.
- Depending on the circumstances, an overspending may not be entirely undesirable.

References

1 Bryans W. *Managing in Health and Social Care: essential checklists for frontline staff.* Oxford: Radcliffe Publishing; 2004.
2 Bryans W. *Resource Management in Health and Social Care: essential checklists.* Oxford: Radcliffe Publishing; 2005. p. 85–86.

Chapter 3

Waste watch: fraud and corruption

The issues

- Whether or not a budget management system is in place there are a number of steps that everyone in health and social care can take to avoid unnecessary losses through fraud and corruption.
- Budget managers should aim to apply the principle of process quality in order to attain these goals.
- This feature is covered extensively in *Managing in Health and Social Care*,[1] but in general it is worth drawing attention to elements such as inexperience, negligence, inaccessible advice or ignorance, which can lead to all sorts of serious wastage problems including the potential for fraud and corruption.
- In order to correct errors and to track down irregularities, unnecessary time and effort has to be allocated and it is likely that there will also be a loss of morale due to the pressure of any subsequent investigation.
- Supply line and financial systems are therefore designed to minimise these incidents.

Introduction

In industry and commerce, losses of 3–5% of turnover are regularly reported. These losses involve a wide spectrum of criminal activity ranging through inventory and other thefts, forgery and bribes.[2] Translated into the public sector, this would be an incredibly high portion of the budget. Yet when we consider that in health and social care facilities, where there are high volumes of traffic and sites are to a large extent open, there is always a regrettable potential for theft.

Also because of the complex nature of health and social care organisations and the effects of constant staff changes, perception of an abnormal situation may be diminished, for example, noticing that cash or a piece of equipment is missing or that a television hasn't actually gone to be repaired.

In health and social care a system or process failure leading to substantial loss is often the way fraud is detected and there are frequent cases of inventory, payroll and other incidents.

Fraud

Fraud is sometimes called 'the white collar crime' because it is so often associated with office workers. Unfortunately it is not restricted to this category of staff and many others, including external suppliers, can be drawn into the criminal scheme. For example, a supplier might submit an invoice for a greater quantity of goods than actually supplied or a trader might deliberately charge more than the agreed price. Of course, health and social care organisations have elaborate and expensive checking arrangements to make sure that this does not happen. But interestingly, some commercial organisations only spot check invoices for small amounts (say £100) because of the high cost of a 100% check. The rest, they pay without query. The problem with this approach is that an unscrupulous trader could submit a large number of invoices for small amounts in the hope that they would not be detected. If they were discovered, the trader could plead an honest mistake.

Where employees are involved, the crime usually requires collusion between at least two employees. Most supply, personnel and finance systems are therefore designed so that the cooperation of two or more members of staff acting independently is required in order to legitimately activate the system.

Basically the fraudster is seeking a loophole through which they can convince the organisation that goods, services, works or staffing were supplied that were not in fact ever delivered. Another type of fraud is when an individual accuses the organisation of being in breach of contract or duty of care for the purpose of financial gain, for example, by claiming for an accidental injury that did not actually happen.

For fraud to be successful, the acquiescence or active participation of the budget manager or a senior member of the department involved in the spending cycle might also be needed. It is therefore the responsibility of everyone (a several responsibility) in the organisation to be alert to the possibility of fraud – that suspicious activity or overtime claim, docket or invoice that does not seem right may be worth another look.

Tips from the front office

- Budget managers who are alert to irregularities are important safeguards against collusion and other irregularities that can occur on the business side of the organisation.
- Encourage and train budget managers or their representatives to provide an independent scrutiny at key purchasing stages in which they have an interest.
- Pay attention to, and where appropriate take action on, other external criticism such as audit comments.

The main points at which a budget or other manager may be involved in a system to prevent collusion and fraud are illustrated in Figure 3.1.

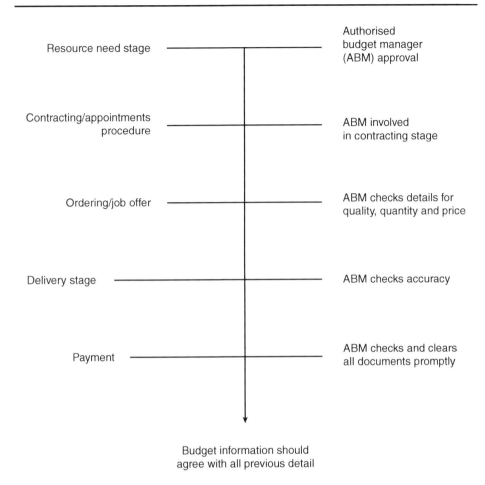

Figure 3.1 shows:

Resource need stage ——————— Authorised budget manager (ABM) approval

Contracting/appointments procedure ——————— ABM involved in contracting stage

Ordering/job offer ——————— ABM checks details for quality, quantity and price

Delivery stage ——————— ABM checks accuracy

Payment ——————— ABM checks and clears all documents promptly

Budget information should agree with all previous detail

Figure 3.1 Elimination stages: collusion in the spending cycle.

Case study

Valerian Grizzle, the newly appointed budget manager for the Near Home Facility, part of the Bigtown Hospital Trust, noticed that the number of staff being charged to her budget exceeded her establishment. She asked for a staff-on-payroll list. From this she confirmed her suspicions. The list included a number of names whose identity was not recognised by anyone else in the facility. She had uncovered a serious fraud whereby salaries were being drawn for non-existent staff and paid into bank accounts eventually traced to a member of the paymaster unit.

Tips from the front office

- Budget overcharging occurs where items unconnected with the particular budget appear as legitimate expenditure.
- Ensure you know and have approved all charges.

- If you are suspicious, inform the appropriate authorities immediately.
- Do not mention or implicate any person or staff member.
- Do not undertake any interviews.
- Do not disturb anything that may be used later as evidence.

Corruption

Corruption originates from sources external to an organisation's due process, for example, the award of contracts and appointments procedures, and occurs where the perpetrator seeks to bring undue influence through gifts, bribes, hospitality, sponsorship or threats, so that the outcome will result in their own illegal gain. The target for this type of activity can be anyone who has influence upon the resource supply chain, including staffing.[3] This type of abuse can range from confusion over a conflict of interest through to the blatant offer of a bribe.

There are, however, a number of steps that can be taken to reduce the chances of corruption.

- Ensure that there are clear instructions available for staff and board members on appropriate behaviour when conducting their legitimate business.
- A strict code of conduct regarding confidentiality should be in place and the organisation's attitude to the serious nature of any breach should be made clear.
- The same code of conduct should be adhered to by any person or commercial organisation seeking to gain confidential information.
- Make sure that employment and contracting are regulated so that documents such as applications and tenders are properly received, recorded and kept safe until they are due to be considered.
- Strictly apply closure dates and times so that no late applicants are ever considered.
- Where tenders are concerned, ensure safe keeping by an independent party and open them in accordance with laid down protocol, recording relevant details at that time.

In this context fraudulent behaviour should not be confused with legitimate gifts, legacies, sponsorship, donations, etc. intended for the direct benefit of patients/clients, as described in *Managing in Health and Social Care*,[4] and which can be enormously beneficial both in terms of goodwill and in situations where normal funding is not possible. However, it has to be stressed that even in those circumstances acceptability criteria have to be established so that sinister influences are discouraged.

On a personal level, those working in clinical areas can be unwitting targets for those who desire to compromise the organisation. The Medicines

(Advertising) Regulations 1994 make it a requirement that no gift, pecuniary advantage or benefit in kind shall be promised, offered or supplied for promotional purposes unless it is inexpensive and relevant. Furthermore it is an offence to solicit any such gift, hospitality or sponsorship prohibited by the Regulations. In order to facilitate the relationship between hospital doctors and commercial interests, The Royal College of Physicians has issued guidelines that define its position on these matters.

General considerations

- **Legality** Make sure offering or accepting the gift does not infringe the law.
- **Ethics** Check that there is no conflict of interest nor damage to integrity.
- **Equity** Test whether the gift is targeted on an individual or group within the organisation.
- **Intention** Be certain that the offer or acceptance of the gift cannot be interpreted as a bribe.

Guidance on promotional schemes

A designated senior manager or director should be made responsible for oversight of schemes such as the following:

- genuine marketing material such as calendars, diaries, pencils, etc. aimed at penetrating the workplace and maintaining existing market connections by creating genuine goodwill
- corporate hospitality to launch or renew interest in a product
- special customers' staff discount schemes
- sponsorship for sporting events and charitable fund-raising.

Acceptability criteria

All organisations should develop guidelines that indicate acceptable limits within which staff must work. These should state:

- when a gift, sponsorship or hospitality can be accepted
- how it shall be accepted
- whether certain items may be retained for the individual's own use
- any other internal procedures.

Tips from the front office

- Maintain a register of all gifts received.
- Donors should always be officially thanked.

- Consider third-party management of funds received.
- Take time to consult on legal, finance, professional and estate matters.
- Ensure you receive regular reports on:
  - progress on purchases and commissioning
  - changes or differences in description
  - all funds held in trust for the department/clinic/practice.

Case study

Dickie Dunders of Dunders, Bashette and Smithers, a well-known local building firm, offered Valerian Grizzle the use of his villa in Spain.

'No strings, Ms Grizzle', he assured her. 'A purely business arrangement.'

As she was a member of the Bigtown Trust Works Contracts sub-group, Ms Grizzle reported the offer.

When confronted, although Dickie Dunders was suitably contrite, he was adamant that Valerian Grizzle had misunderstood the offer. He said that he had meant that if she accepted the offer, he expected payment.

Key point summary

- Health and social care organisations are not exempt from fraud and corruption.
- These are hidden costs and unnecessary burdens on already over-stretched budgets which should be eliminated.
- Where there are loopholes in the system or where staff do not pay attention to business details, then exploitation of those weaknesses can take place.
- Budget managers and their staff have a several responsibility to be alert to the existence of 'white-collar crime'.
- Clear instructions should be made available to all those conducting business on behalf of their organisation, especially in connection with the acceptance of gifts and hospitality.
- As with patients/clients, care should be taken to ensure business confidentiality.
- Irregularities, especially those contained in audit reports, must be taken seriously and corrective action implemented.
- Budget managers and staff must be suitably briefed so that they know how to deal with suspected incidents.

References

1 Bryans W. *Managing in Health and Social Care: essential checklists for frontline staff.* Oxford: Radcliffe Publishing; 2004. Chapter 1.
2 *Ibid.* Chapter 3.
3 *Ibid.* Chapter 5.
4 *Ibid.* Chapter 2.

Chapter 4

Waste watch: reducing other losses

The issues

- Within every budget manager's domain, there are key areas where waste and loss of resources are a daily occurrence.
- The contracting-supply-payment system provides enormous scope for the unnecessary creation of loss.
- But with the cooperation and active participation of the budget manager, it is possible to keep losses to a minimum.
- Their prevention is not dependent upon budgetary management.
- Losses are obvious if managers and other key staff are active and alert to possible weak points.
- In order to avoid process failure, it is imperative that budget managers and key frontline staff who generate spending at all levels ensure that relevant protocols and deadlines are both observed and consistently implemented.
- This chapter identifies four key areas where managers and their staff can achieve these goals through an ordered process.
  - Improve the security of resources.
  - Maximise financial process quality.
  - Improve staff morale.
  - Reduce any abuse of resources.

Improve the security of resources

There are a variety of motives for theft and pilfering. These include low morale, poor pay and succumbing to a challenge. But lax control provides constant opportunity and temptation, which managers and other staff must identify and minimise.

Much of the detail required in internal supplies, personnel and financial systems, although potentially tedious to supply, is designed to minimise the opportunity for theft and pilfering. However, the success of such systems depends on the accuracy, compliance and determination of managers and their staff to ensure that what is being paid for was:

- needed in the first place
- properly authorised and within budget
- officially ordered or contracted
- received in good condition and at the right quality and quantity
- in the case of equipment, properly commissioned, made suitable for use and properly secured
- in the case of new staff, properly inducted, trained and deployed.

When resources have been delivered on site, as long as there is no mechanism to provide security, they are vulnerable to theft and pilfering. The main targets are those that facilitate easy transportation and conversion into cash, including cash itself. These aspects have been extensively covered in *Managing in Health and Social* Care,[1] but because theft can affect the organisation, staff and patients/clients, it is worth reiterating the key features relating to the security of cash.

Don't

- Take cash from strangers. Be polite, but find out the business of the potential benefactor and anticipate a hidden and unethical agenda.
- Accept a gift for an unrealistic purpose.
- Accept a personal gift or act on behalf of a colleague.
- Keep cash in insecure receptacles such as desk drawers or filing cabinets.

Do

- Observe strict rules about keys to secure places.
- Count cash in the presence of the benefactor or a witness.
- Keep a record.
- Write a receipt.
- Make regular lodgements.
- Ensure an official letter of thanks is dispatched.
- Make sure you receive regular reports on accumulated funds.
- Maintain the right to influence spending.

Tips from the front office

- Treat cash with respect.
- Think of cash as being too hot to handle.
- Regard cash as a dangerous substance.

Maximise financial process quality

Frontline clinical or social service budget managers consume resources for the improvement in patients'/clients' conditions whereas service or support departments, such as payroll, provide essential and fundamental benefits to staff. This is illustrated in Figure 4.1.

It is my experience that losses occur where there is a loophole in the system, where, because of other pressures, a manager has not properly supervised what must seem to be mundane tasks or where a more relaxed attitude has crept into a particular culture.

In their drive to minimise waste, financial managers can unwittingly create the perception that the integrity of other departments is being constantly scrutinised. This damages an important interdependency with budget managers. In order to reduce losses and waste, supply-line and

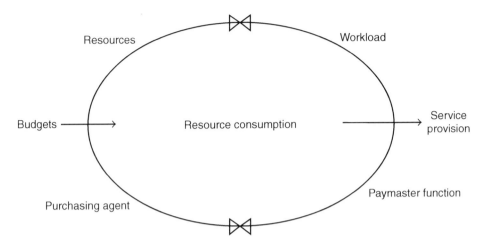

Figure 4.1   Resource management process.

financial process quality assurance require the vigilance, active participation and involvement of the budget manager, especially where exceptions
and irregular features such as overtime require compliance with finance-
led deadlines. The consistent missing of deadlines by the budget manager,
whether through ignorance, negligence or non-compliance, can lead to
losses.

- Late payment of overtime will cause resentment on the part of the
  staff concerned and will also produce inaccurate budget statements.
- Discounts can be lost if the claim time has lapsed.
- Late reporting of the non-delivery or short delivery of expected
  goods can lead to the carrier refusing to accept responsibility.

Co-operation, rather than deadlock, through agreed protocols is essential.

- Maximum use of, and reasonable access to, staff at control points,
  characterised by the various events in the supply or payment
  chains must be agreed.
- Where deficiencies have been detected as a result of audit, review or
  other techniques, budget managers need to be amenable to any necessary investigation – they need to understand the significant factors
  and cooperate.
- Communications relating to budgetary, costing, statistical or other
  performance indicators must be made part of an ongoing dialogue.
- New performance initiatives should be agreed with heads of department before commencement.
- Responsibilities and authorities must be defined for accountability
  purposes.
- Rather than forcing every issue to the top of the office, realistic contact points for routine dialogue with the budget managers should be
  established further down the hierarchical chain.

- Finance managers need to convince budget managers that their role is ever helpful.

Tips from the front office

- Keep relations with heads of other departments on a professional basis.
- Make sure all your data and other facts are accurate before you engage in communication. Ask more than once, can this be right? And check it again! Failure to do so can damage your credibility.

Case study

During a special audit carried out before Valerian Grizzle took up post in the Near Home Facility, it was discovered that her predecessor had saved money on the payroll budget by delaying the submission of overtime and other special payment claims. This would have to be corrected during Ms Grizzle's tenure without the addition of extra funds, resulting in budget overspend. (*See* Figure 4.2 for the effects.) The treasurer told her that there would doubtless be savings from improved morale and these would help compensate.

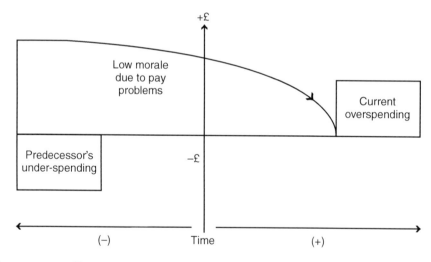

Figure 4.2   Effects of delayed payments.

Twelve steps to improve morale and reduce losses

Improving staff morale is at the core of good management. It becomes dynamic when the right incentives and discipline are used to stimulate and generate action through motivation and leadership. But who or what makes people work, work harder or even work for nothing? Theories abound, but it is generally accepted that motivational drives lie within the complex needs–wants–satisfaction chain reaction and are the basic stimuli that induce activity. However, gratification of all the disparate workforce drives would be an impossible management task: some moderation is necessary. Conversely, in times of crisis such as war people will work for nothing more than 'blood, sweat and tears' – equitable treatment, discipline and hope of an improvement are possible common denominators.

From earliest times, morale has been generally recognised as one of the key factors that facilitate or diminish an organisation's capacity to be successful. And many of the causes of poor budget performance can be traced back to the indifference of overworked, transient staff who may have little or no commitment to the particular department or unit to which they have been allocated.

The ability to recognise and improve poor or low morale is therefore an essential management attribute and taking proper measures will enhance performance. Below are 12 steps aimed at creating the conditions for improvement.

Create a stable workforce

In the context of creating an awareness of waste and loss, a constantly changing, dissatisfied workforce is counterproductive mainly because of the difficulties of generating enthusiasm through team effort and therefore an awareness of potential weaknesses.

Establish a performance database

A common reason given for poor performance is that morale is low. Indeed, 'couldn't care less, I've enough to do' attitudes are often at the centre of many losses suffered in health and social care. But without some definitive measurements it is impossible to establish whether morale really is low or not.

Certainly, worrying levels of accidents, complaints, negligence, mistakes, fraud, deliberate vandalism, etc. linked to one department or workplace would indicate that something is wrong, but if the underlying reasons appear to be connected with heavy workloads that are underpinned by various types of absenteeism and high rates of staff turnover, then appropriate further investigation and action need to be taken.

Keep records of high turnover rates, sickness, absenteeism and any other untoward events; obtain comparisons from similar departments and/or other organisations. Keep records of disciplinary matters. Assess the state of morale based upon reliable data.

Clear and achievable objectives

Conflicting or, taking account of resource levels, impossible objectives diminish morale. Ensure a sense of direction, give and get commitment – agreed mission statements are often efficacious.

Discipline

Make sure the organisation's code of conduct is reasonable, appropriate and acceptable and that it is applied impartially.

Process quality

Foster a culture of doing the right thing first time, every time.

Foster departmental pride

Generate pride in work performed through team working and the provision of team figures for productivity and market share. Encourage ideas for general improvement and for developments that will lead to expansion of patient/client benefits.

Equality

Ensure that all employees, from the bottom to the top, are treated with equal respect and are paid according to the work they do, not who or what they are.

Conditions of employment

As well as rewards and remuneration, conditions can be systematically improved by enhancing the working environment so that it is appropriate to the tasks undertaken. Health and safety, cleanliness, lighting, heat, decoration, state of repair, canteen and toilet facilities, are simple considerations that affect workforce morale.

Awkward customer relations

High customer/client expectation, coupled with the frustration of dealing with a large and apparently impersonal organisation, has in recent years produced the customer rage phenomenon. Staff who have to deal with such difficulties may suffer a loss of morale and management must take a proactive role in providing support.

Training

Induction and ongoing training programmes are important assets in the drive to improve morale. Make sure that feelings and complaints expressed in the classroom are properly channelled into the system so their impact can be assessed.

Communication

An open system of communication and information will help dispel any adverse rumours or at least will facilitate the management of bad news.

Developing the human organisation

Evolving structures tend to take on characteristics of their own and have a deep impact on workforce performance. In sophisticated cases, organisations are perceived to have their own culture, ethics, symbols and market reputation with which staff identify. In the best and simplest examples, staff must have adequate rewards, job satisfaction, prospects and a sense of security. Training programmes and involvement are essential to building an effective communication network with staff.

Tips from the front office

A plan to tackle waste, based on a survey of the above factors converted into acceptability criteria, can be readily drawn up but its implementation needs to be measured against databases and observations so that a genuine increase in morale is seen to be matched by improvements in productivity.

Reduce any abuse of resources

There are a number of factors that lead to the abuse and therefore waste of resources. Mainly because of the responsive nature of our services, these factors can operate without managers being aware of having made a conscious decision. Four examples are listed below.

Workload

The consistent overwork of resources (in whichever category they fall, including staff) will eventually put them beyond a point of toleration, resulting in unnecessary repairs, replacements and the filling of an increased number of vacancies. This will be the obvious part of the cost of such abuse. It is better to establish limits beyond which resources will not be extended and, where appropriate, previously agreed numbers could be used for this purpose.

Health and safety

Often, reductions in the use of resources are made in the interests of economy, such as lowering the levels of heat and light. Such action may actually create new hazards and if an accident happens as a result, any original savings will have been counterproductive.

Time

As a finite resource, time, and how it is used, are crucial elements in both resource and budget management. However, as part of any service provision it is imperative to allocate a certain amount of time so that contingencies can readily be dealt with. There are many areas, such as the constant use of the telephone, unnecessary meetings,[2] attendance at conferences and courses, where savings in time can be made.

Space

The effective and efficient use of the space provided is an important aspect of waste control. Clearly, if clutter is allowed to accumulate, it is a hazard and is wasting space that could be better utilised. It is important to ensure that valuable space is not devoted to stockpiling and budget managers should make sure they use supply lines to guarantee just-in-time deliveries (JIT)[3] so that special requirements can be suitably reduced.

Key point summary

- Be particular when specifying the need for new or replacement resources.
- Fit and develop a budget plan around your requirements.
- Identify sources and prices.
- Allocate a budget or make a bid for additional monies.
- Participate in the negotiation and contracting process.
- Ensure that the methods for receiving and/or inducting resources are secure and that sophisticated equipment is properly commissioned and maintained.
- Clear all documents in accordance with agreed deadlines.
- Make sure that vulnerable and easily transportable resources like cash are properly secured.
- Promote the efficient and effective management of resources within your domain.

References

1 Bryans W. *Managing in Health and Social Care: essential checklists for frontline staff.* Oxford: Radcliffe Publishing; 2004. Chapter 3.
2 Bryans W. How to chair effective meetings. *Health Management.* 2006; **March/April**: 29.
3 Bryans W. How to get the most from the supply chain. *Health Management.* 2005; **July/August**: 29.

Chapter 5

What is a budget?

The issues

- Budget definitions are often confusing. For example, we may mean money when we talk about resources or we can mean a prescribed quantity of materials or number of staff instead of actual funds. For a number of reasons connected with the way spending is managed, these are not always interchangeable.
- At whatever level and whether they are operating in commissioner or provider mode, budget managers purchase or commission resources for consumption within their internal environment and provide enhanced benefit, value-added goods and services, care and treatment to their external environments.
- A budget is a set amount of money or a ration of resources allocated to an authorised manager for a specific purpose and intended to cover a defined period of time.[1]
- Sometimes it is also the description of an organisation's total funds, which may be expressed as a single amount or as a comprehensive list of individual budgets.
- Methods of budget calculation may vary and spending patterns will fluctuate, but it is essential that at all levels in the organisation, there is an underlying comprehension and agreement on what is expected.
- It follows that a flow of relevant and accurate information should be established by which performance is interpreted and measured, appropriate intervention is taken and future activity is planned.
- Generally speaking, there are two ways of reporting performance. One examines spending against a target and reports the variation; the other subtracts total spending from the total amount available and reports what is left.
- This chapter examines the basic principles of budgetary management in the context of the internal environment and looks at differing requirements when managing once-and-for-all expenditure as opposed to the continuity of day-to-day demands.

Introduction: the purposes of budget management

The main purpose of budget management in health and social care is to provide an early indication of resource performance within the limits of time and money so that, if necessary, appropriate intervention is possible.

Budget management in health and social care is made possible through a process whereby both spending authority and responsibility are delegated to those managers deemed best placed to maintain a spending discipline. The system that facilitates this process is a management tool that signals deviations from an agreed target and enables any remedial action to be taken in time.

With the emphasis firmly on spending controls and appropriate interventions, it follows that the reporting system has to be as near to real time as possible – retrospective or historical analysis will not do. This implies simplicity rather than complexity. It also demands competent and accountable budget managers.

Broadly speaking, most budget management systems have three main benefits. They assist the individual to manage within agreed limits, provide a coordinating function to both the organisation and the individual manager, and facilitate the organisation as a whole to make realistic decisions on both tactical and strategic levels. Collectively, these features support planning and forecasting and provide a structure for the reconciliation of service requirements with limited resources so that the needs of patients/clients are considered in a rational framework.

As budgets are inevitably based on the type and number of resources required to undertake particular tasks, there is often a dilemma concerning the way in which systems will report on performance.

Money and/or rations

A budget may be expressed in terms of a resource ration,[1] for example, as so many staff in a ward to undertake a particular task, the number of people in an office to cope with bureaucracy, the number of theatre packs needed for certain procedures, community staff commensurate with dependency, portion control in the staff restaurant, etc.

Expressing a budget as a package of money can seem to be a more attractive format. This is mainly because the purchase and consumption of resources can be rationalised and recorded in this commonly understood medium, but also because it is more easily accessible as a general method of measurement and comparison. However, the utilisation of expenditure as a uniform mode of communication also has its problems because there are distinctive spending patterns associated with different aspects of service delivery. For example, there must be a distinction between capital expenditure, which is reserved for new, once only, large, expensive items such as buildings and major items of equipment and revenue expenditure, which is mainly spending on day-to-day or ongoing commitments like payroll, drugs, materials and other goods and services. Within the revenue headings there are also distinctions between payroll, which accounts for 80%+ of day-to-day expenditure, and goods and services spending, which includes repairs and replacements of drugs and medical and surgical equipment.

There is a further complication pertaining to revenue expenditure that does not conform to a regular pattern, for example, overtime, sickness, holiday relief, replacement furniture and equipment, and maintenance contracts. Because budget payroll systems, which can account for over 80% of revenue spending, have grown ever more sophisticated it is now customary to indicate the quantity of resources the allocated amount of money will buy. Thus it is not unusual to discover payroll budgets expressed as a combination of rations and money. Surprisingly, this can lead to more confusion than if they had been expressed in a unitary way.

Some of the problems are illustrated in the following case study.

Case study

Valerian Grizzle, a newly appointed project manager for community liaison and support at the Bigtown Hospital Trust, had a budget allocation of £1.2m. According to the documentation, this was the equivalent of 60 staff.

In a memo to Midas Luckpenny, the treasurer, she noted that this averaged out at £20k per person, but early expenditure trends were very erratic and seemed to indicate that she could afford more staff (*see* Figure 5.1).

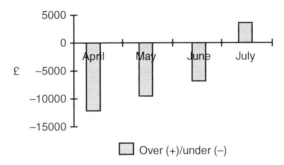

Figure 5.1 Budget variations for the first four months.

Time frames

Because of the need for reassurance that money and/or resources will not run out, budgets and time periods are inextricably linked.

A budget, whether it is an allocation of money or a ration of resources, is always limited by time – a week, a month, a year or longer. Because most budgets must be made to last the distance, managers need to know the time span that the budget is intended to cover. If, however, the budget is for a once-and-for-all project like capital expenditure, then usually it does not much matter when it is exhausted, as long as it is spent within the time frame and the project is completed on time and within budget, unless there are other factors to consider. This is dealt with in more detail from Chapter 6 onwards.

Where a budget is for continuous expenditure such as payroll, the budget must be divided out over the number of weeks/months that are in the period so that performance can be measured and appropriate steps taken to correct an undesirable situation. However, it is usual for even apparently simple budgets to have an element of complexity, which will cause expenditure patterns to fluctuate over the whole period. For example, changes in weather, unexpected surges of sickness, non-delivery of resources, staff and other shortages can all cause fluctuations. Generally some sort of contingency arrangements are built into the budget to cover these situations, but it is also important that budget managers do not become confused over the distinctions. In this context, the project manager in the case study needed some urgent guidance; otherwise she might have made a serious error of judgement.

Case study

Midas Luckpenny replied to Valerian Grizzle stating that from the total amount she should allow a contingency reserve of approximately 12.5% or £150k for sickness and holiday relief staff. This would leave £1.05m to be spread evenly over the year in equal segments of £87,500 per month. The reserve of £150k should be added in as relief staff were taken on until the reserve was exhausted.

Simple budget profiles

There are two simple profiles, which are the result of the division between longer-term expenditure like capital and day-to-day revenue expenditure or running costs. Figure 5.2 is intended to eliminate any confusion brought about by the overlap of longer-term spending into the revenue portion.

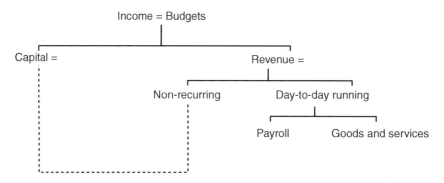

Figure 5.2 Income and expenditure divisions.

The profile is arrived at by deciding how the budget is to be reported. Should the budget be divided into 52 or 12 equal segments according to the frequency of spend and reported each week or each month as a simple variation? Or should it be adjusted each week or month to reflect changing circumstances and if so, how would control of the budget be maintained?

With capital spending, longer-term revenue expenditure and the management of projects, even though spending is planned and orders placed, there is always a distinct possibility of delay at the outset and the likely irregularity of delivery of supplies. Irregularity also occurs with certain types of payroll expenditure like holiday and sickness relief or overtime. This means that splitting the budget into equal segments spread over the financial year will produce considerable fluctuations that are difficult to interpret.

An example is shown in Table 5.1, where a capital budget of £100k has been split into equal segments over the time period. While the total budget was notified at the beginning of the year, it has taken to the third month for goods to arrive and they have continued to do so on an irregular basis (in financial terms). This means that splitting the budget into 12 equal segments of £8,333 per month has resulted in a totally inaccurate assessment of the true position and any ill-informed observer of the first two months' performance would conclude that there was £16,700 in hand, whereas that amount has clearly been committed and the whole budget will be spent by the end of the year. The degree of variation using this method is illustrated in Figure 5.3.

Table 5.1   Sample capital budget and spending

Month	Over/under	Budget £k	Expenditure £k
April	−8.3	8.3	0
May	−8.3	8.3	0
June	1.6	8.4	10
July	3.7	8.3	12
August	0.7	8.3	9
September	4.6	8.4	13
October	3.7	8.3	12
November	1.7	8.3	10
December	0.6	8.4	9
January	−0.3	8.3	8
February	0.7	8.3	9
March	−0.4	8.4	8
		100	100

There is an interesting comparison between this type of performance and that illustrated in Figure 5.1, where within Valerian Grizzle's total budget a significant amount for sickness and holiday relief was not amenable to division into equal parts.

Where spending is expected to be irregular it has been shown that reporting a variation might be difficult to interpret. In these cases reporting is best undertaken on a cumulative basis whilst at the same time giving the balance remaining unspent so that the budget manager can control the budget more readily. Table 5.2 and Figure 5.4 illustrate this type of profile.

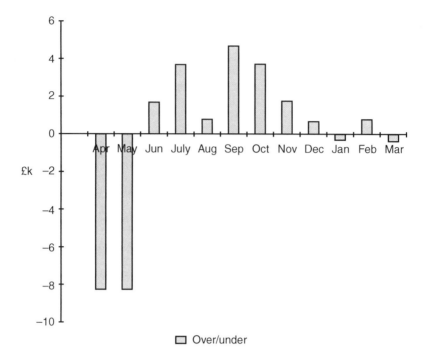

Figure 5.3   Capital spending variations.

Table 5.2   Balance remaining on capital budget

Month	Expenditure (£k)	Cumulative (£k)	Budget remainder (£k)
April	0		100
May	0		100
June	10	10	90
July	12	22	78
August	9	31	69
September	13	44	56
October	12	56	44
November	10	66	34
December	9	75	25
January	8	83	17
February	9	92	8
March	8	100	0

Calculating the budget target in accordance with the profile

As explained above, it is important to segregate all the component parts in deciding what the weekly/monthly target is to be. Some of these will be equal amounts for each time period where the spending is more or less

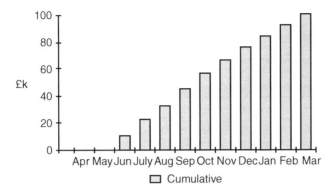

Figure 5.4 Capital spending profile.

predictable. Others will be subject to ad hoc arrangements according to the budget manager's local knowledge or some agreed protocol with the finance department. Thus the original supposition by the project manager in our example was based on an incorrect calculation of the budget target, as illustrated in Table 5.3. The adjusted budget targets are illustrated in Table 5.4.

Table 5.3   Incorrect budget calculation

Months	Monthly spend (£)	Monthly target (£)	Over	Under
April	87,500	100,000		12,500
May	90,000	100,000		10,000
June	92,500	100,000		7,500
July	102,500	100,000	2,500	

Table 5.4   Adjusted budget targets

Months	Relief budget (£)	Monthly target (£)	Total
April		87,500	87,500
May	2,500	87,500	90,000
June	5,000	87,500	92,500
July	15,000	87,500	102,500
Cumulatives	22,500	350,000	372,500
Total budget	150,000	1,050,000	1,200,000
Remainders	127,500	700,000	827,500

Case study

Midas Luckpenny pointed out that in deciding the amount to be added in from her reserve, Valerian Grizzle appeared simply to have taken the difference between her basic budget and expenditure. The result of this calculation was that she was neither over- nor underspent. In his view, this would be a very unusual situation if it were true. Valerian Grizzle argued that she still had £127,500 in reserve.

Table 5.5   Significant variations throughout the year

Months	Monthly spend (£)	Cumulative (£)
April	8,750	8,750
May	9,000	17,750
June	9,250	27,000
July	10,250	37,250
August	12,250	49,500
September	10,250	59,750
October	9,000	68,750
November	8,750	77,500
December	9,500	87,000
January	10,500	97,500
February	10,750	108,250
March	11,750	120,000
Total	120,000	

Key point summary

- Nowadays, most budgets are expressed in money terms, but they often incorporate supporting data that show the items that could be or have been purchased.
- For simplicity, budgets can be divided into two basic types. Those that are frequently and almost equally occurring, for example, basic payroll, are called regularly occurring budgets. Budgets intended for infrequent spending, for example, equipment, works, some forms of payroll, etc., are called non-recurring budgets.
- We can create a simple budget profile according to the type of budget we want to manage. Here are the basic steps.
  - Calculate, by referring to historical patterns, the amount required for regularly occurring expenditure, the basic payroll elements, the regular goods and services payments, store withdrawals, etc.
  - Examine the list of non-recurring items, prioritise competing demands and balance with the remainder.
  - At this juncture, it is also worth putting aside a contingency reserve to cover exceptional and unexpected demands.
  - Re-examine as appropriate and approve non-recurring demands.

- Divide the total money available for the particular period into the appropriate categories, making sure that it balances.
- Take the recurring budget and apportion it equally over the period according to the number of discernible segments, for example, the annual total of weekly wages would be apportioned week by week.
- Keep back the non-recurring portion, adding it in only as specific expenditure occurs.

Reference

1 Bryans W. *Resource Management in Health and Social Care: essential checklists.* Oxford: Radcliffe Publishing; 2005.

Chapter 6

Profiling and managing budgets

The issues

In specific circumstances, it is essential that budget managers become familiar with the intricacies of emerging spending patterns so that they can immediately recognise an irregularity. This knowledge can be gleaned from the following sources:

- historical data where records of similar situations indicate an important lesson on the way expenditure is likely to progress, for example, those budgets that are linked to seasonal variations or are fixed in accordance with priorities such as a capital allocation
- personal experience or experience that has been passed on can contain valuable lessons
- changes generated by the manager/management, which should be part of a financial plan in which peaks and troughs will already have been identified.

Budget managers who are able to identify unexpected fluctuations can more quickly source the cause (which might in the long run be found to be legitimate) and hopefully will be able to correct the situation. The benefits of this are to be able to:

- amend incorrect data
- initiate early action on management issues relating to resource consumption
- identify irregularities that might be caused by attempted fraud or theft.

Introduction

In addition to the simple distinction in the profiles of recurring and non-recurring expenditure, there are a number of other spending events that are contrary to the expected normal appearance. These are caused either by fairly obvious factors such as seasonal variations through to spikes in expenditure resulting from major unexpected incidents such as the sudden failure of expensive diagnostic or surgical equipment.

Some of these events are amenable to the creation of a budget profile that will nearly mirror spending behaviour, for example, for budgets in the heat, power and lighting category. Other budgets, such as those that are demand-responsive and generally appear to be casual expenditure, are more difficult to manage. In these cases it is usual to keep a small contingency reserve against unexpected surges in spending.

Sometimes, in exceptional circumstances, an additional allocation may be made available for untoward events. In these situations, budget managers need to be alert to the possibility of having to make a bid for additional resources. This aspect was extensively dealt with in *Managing in Health and Social Care*.[1]

Situations that have been contrived by the budget manager are in a different category. In all circumstances, it is important to tailor the budget profile to reflect the changes being made internally. This is particularly relevant where there is an alteration in the balance of care in which specific service is contracting, thus resulting in reductions in the budget amount. The opposite situation occurs where there are developments. Then budget managers need to ensure that the agreed additional funding is added to their profiles at appropriate moments. In common with the spending behaviour in both retraction and development circumstances, changes in the pattern of workloads can also have detrimental or beneficial effects on the spending pattern.

Casual or demand-responsive expenditure

There are many types of demand-responsive budget and this category can cover special purposes like unforeseen irreparable breakdown and other charges such as unexpected maintenance. An illustration of the apparently casual nature of this type of spending is shown in Figure 6.1.

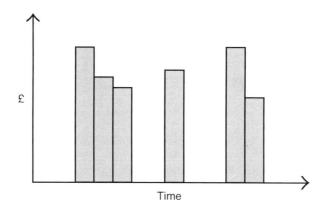

Figure 6.1 Casual expenditure.

The emerging pattern can range through a continuous flow of erratic spending, to an all-at-once commitment to major expenditure that can happen at any juncture in the financial period. Other examples that have already been mentioned include holiday and sickness relief staff, some training budgets, minor replacements of plant, machinery, furniture and equipment, and some repairs.

Infrequent but predictable expenditure

Included in this budget category are those charges that are fixed and where the incidence is known, for example, extra bank holiday payments. *See* Figure 6.2. Although charges occur at apparently irregular intervals, they are in fact already known to the budget manager. Take holiday pay, for example: as well as extra bank holiday payments, numerous other areas have to be included.

- Sickness and holiday relief expenditure will occur in accordance with this type of expenditure.
- Cleansing and special cleaning operations may be scheduled for holiday periods.
- Certain remedial works and refurbishments may be planned around times when workloads are slack.
- Some waiting list initiatives and day surgery may have this kind of impact upon expenditure.

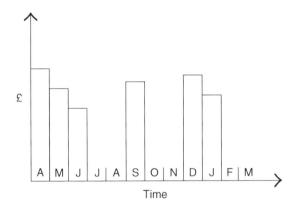

Figure 6.2   Infrequent predictable expenditure.

Seasonally responsive budgets

The use of seasonally responsive budget profiles is appropriate where there is a distinct but gradual variation that occurs according to the time of year. And while budgets for heat, power and light are obvious candidates, other budgets such as sickness relief may also be profiled in this way. Figure 6.3 illustrates a heating budget. Interestingly, this type of profile also suits certain drug consumption where drugs are used specifically to treat seasonally influenced diseases.

In contrast, the effects of sudden phenomena such as weather hazards in winter can be obtained for the number of patients/clients visited in the community. Although it is impossible to accurately predict the weather, this method does provide a better guideline than simply dividing the annual budget by 12. An example is given in the sample budget statement in Table 6.1.

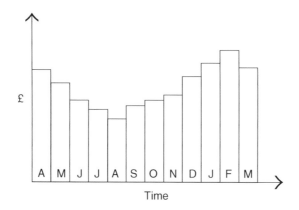

Figure 6.3   Profiled heating budget.

Table 6.1   Heat, power and light budget for Near Home Facility: year's performance compared with the profile

Months	Budget (£)	Expenditure (£)	Over/under (£)
April	9,000	10,000	1,000
May	8,000	7,000	−1,000
June	6,000	4,000	−2,000
July	5,000	7,000	2,000
August	4,000	5,000	1,000
September	5,000	6,000	1,000
October	6,000	7,000	1,000
November	7,000	8,000	1,000
December	8,000	9,000	1,000
January	10,000	7,000	−3,000
February	12,000	12,000	0
March	9,000	10,000	1,000
Totals	89,000	92,000	3,000

On the other hand, if equal segments had been used to give a monthly budget of approximately £7,400 per month, the erratic nature of the variations would be as illustrated in Table 6.2.

Table 6.2 Comparison of results

Months	Equal segments (£)	Expenditure (£)	Simple variation (£)	Original +/– (£)
April	7,400	10,000	2,600	1,000
May	7,400	7,000	−400	−1,000
June	7,400	4,000	−3,400	−2,000
July	7,400	7,000	−400	2,000
August	7,400	5,000	−2,400	1,000
September	7,400	6,000	−1,400	1,000
October	7,400	7,000	−400	1,000
November	7,400	8,000	600	1,000
December	7,400	9,000	1,600	1,000
January	7,400	7,000	−400	−3,000
February	7,400	12,000	4,600	0
March	7,600	10,000	2,400	1,000
Totals	89,000	92,000	3,000	3,000

This is graphically shown in Figure 6.4.

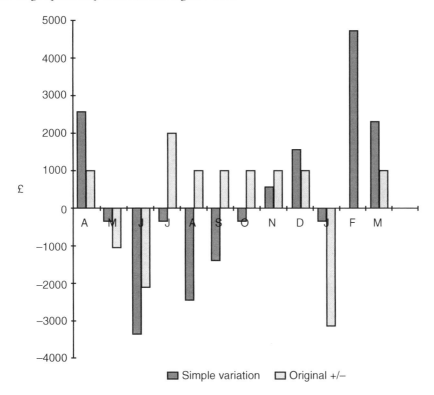

Figure 6.4 Comparison of variations.

The differences between the two methods and the clear benefits of a system using a profile is shown on a cumulative basis in Table 6.3 and graphically in Figure 6.5.

Table 6.3 Relative accuracy of profiled budget

Months	Cumulative simple variation (£)	Cumulative original +/– (£)
April	2,600	1,000
May	2,200	0
June	−1,200	−2,000
July	−1,600	0
August	−400	1,000
September	−5,400	2,000
October	−5,800	3,000
November	−5,200	4,000
December	−3,600	5,000
January	−400	2,000
February	600	2,000
March	3,000	3,000

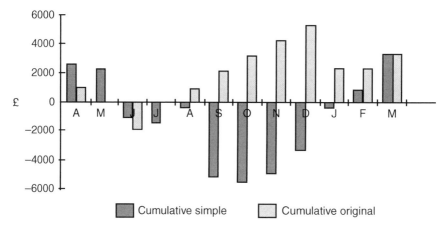

Figure 6.5 Graphic representation of profile accuracy.

Although the profiled budget results have variations, they are in fact signalling at an early stage that the budget is going overspent. Equal segmentation results in quite wild fluctuations that are accurate only in the last month.

Interestingly, if a variation occurs on a well-defined profile, leaving aside any adjustments that might have to be made for exceptionally inclement weather, it should be investigated.

Case study

The heating oil budget for the Near Home Facility showed an unexpected downturn in June, but in July the situation was reversed. There was no reasonable explanation as July's temperature was very much lower. An investigation revealed that an invoice for a delivery in late June had not been included until July. This is illustrated in Figure 6.6.

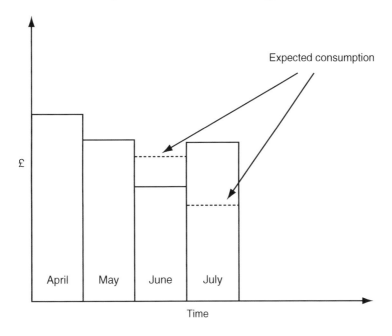

Figure 6.6   Heating oil consumption in Near Home Facility.

When a similarly unexpected large peak occurred in December, at first it was thought that again an invoice from the previous period had been paid late. This profile is illustrated in Figure 6.7, which shows the rate of consumption for the whole year.

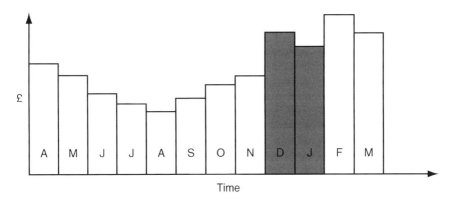

Figure 6.7   Annual oil consumption in Near Home Facility.

However, it turned out that this was not the case and, after further investigation, it appeared that at least two fills of oil had been received during December, which had not been supervised. It was concluded therefore that the unit had been 'overcharged'. There was no proof of any wrong-doing, but a stricter regime for subsequent deliveries was implemented.

Retraction profile

Most readers will be familiar with the variety of quirky savings schemes such as 'efficiency savings'. There are an equal number of quirky responses such as reducing administration, energy savings and finding more efficient ways of working. All these are hard to pin down and possibly ignore the connection between workload and budget. This feature was dealt with in *Resource Management in Health and Social Care*.[2]

However, in order to achieve changes in service delivery and sometimes simply to live in reduced circumstances, it is necessary to make identifiable amendments to service delivery that accommodate the reduction. The expected profile for these schemes is illustrated in Figure 6.8. The main objective is to meet the savings target within the time limit. But, as previously discussed, although delay is inevitable for planning and consultative purposes, it greatly reduces the capacity to achieve the degree of resource shedding necessary to meet the desired target.

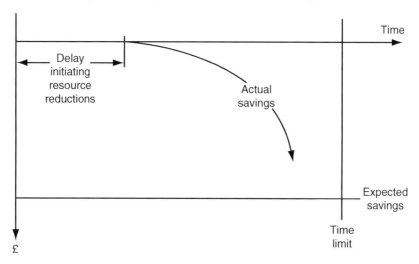

Figure 6.8   Reducing budget profile.

Development situations

Expenditure profiles in connection with improvements and developments reflect the popularity of this type of budget management. This is illustrated in Figure 6.9.

In this category (which may confusingly also include items mentioned under casual profiles above) are items in slightly longer-term once-and-for-all spending such as capital, non-recurring revenue and expenditure arising from the management of projects including IT.

The shape is characterised by a deceptively low or no expenditure record in the early stages followed by a rapidly accelerating trend towards the end of the period, hopefully until the target is reached. Tables 5.1 and 5.2 and Figures 5.3 and 5.4 also help to illustrate the detail of this type of profile.

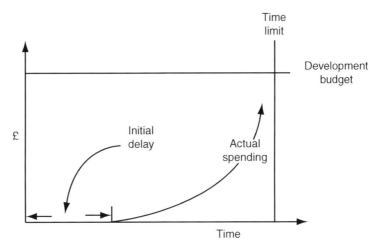

Figure 6.9 Development profile.

Introduction to development control

Although spending development money is more attractive than having to reduce a service in order to make savings, controlling spending within the limits agreed is just as difficult. Potential problems result from two factors (illustrated in Figure 6.10):

- delay at the outset in obtaining deliveries and making payments
- the gap which opens up between items to which we are committed through contracts and other devices and the actual payments, which of necessity lag behind.

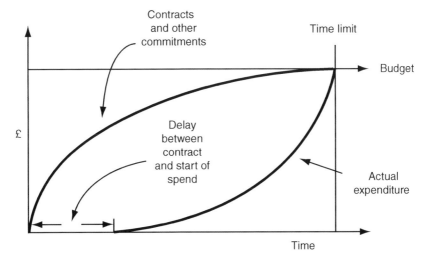

Figure 6.10 Controlling developments.

The main methods for controlling this situation are:

- constant review of the amount that has been committed and the amount that has been paid (the difference between the contracts and other commitments curve and the actual expenditure curve)
- the budget balance that is still available to be spent (the difference between the commitment curve and the total budget target).

As the time limit expires, critical decisions relating to whether certain commitments will be delivered in time have to be balanced against possible overspending, taken together with other emerging priorities.

Pure running expenses

Once the whole spectrum of irregular budget behaviour has been distilled out of the total budget, in theory, the remainder, which represents pure running expenses, should perform each week and each month on an almost equal basis. The profile for this type of activity, which represents the bulk of the budget, would therefore conform with equal segmentation, as illustrated in Figure 6.11 (a rare situation where both budget and spending are perfectly matched).

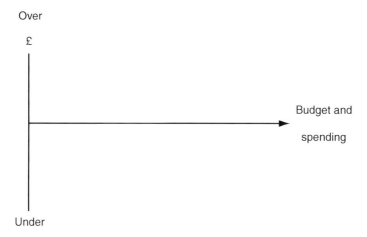

Figure 6.11 Running expenses profile.

Key point summary

- The creation of a budget profile for specific purposes helps managers to separate out those budgetary elements whose spending trends do not behave or are likely not to conform to a regular pattern.
- This enables a predetermined variable budget target to be applied over the weeks and months of the accounting period.
- This exercise should leave the bulk of a recurring or running expenses budget to be managed on an incremental basis.

- When compared with actual expenditure trends, budget profiles are important indicators of irregularities.

References

1 Bryans W. *Managing in Health and Social Care: essential checklists for frontline staff.* Oxford: Radcliffe Publishing; 2004. p. 87–91.
2 Bryans W. *Resource Management in Health and Social Care: essential checklists.* Oxford: Radcliffe Publishing; 2005. Chapter 5.

Chapter 7

How budget management should work

The issues

- Persistent overspending on health and social care budgets means that eventually there will be no money left to pay the wages, salaries and other outgoings.
- In the commercial world, unless some rescue package was put together, this would lead to a firm's liquidation.
- When there are serious shortcomings a similar dilemma faces health and social services managers.
- Conversely, although a rarer occurrence, underspendings can be equally worrying because they indicate an underlying inability to attain or acquire the physical and human resources needed to provide the relevant service.
- There is an expectation that in financial terms effective budget management will deliver books that balance.
- It is widely accepted that this process is most effective when suitable managers at local level are identified, to whom both the responsibility and authority for spending are delegated.
- But there are a number of organisational issues, together with the temptation to impose too many rules, that can impair success.
- In order to make an arrangement work, it is imperative that frequent and accurate information on progress is made available within timescales that facilitate tactical intervention.
- And it follows that when this information is received, it is properly scrutinised by the local manager and that, where appropriate, corrective action is taken.

Introduction

There are a number of factors that influence the effectiveness of budgetary management systems. Some of these were touched upon in both *Managing in Health and Social Care*[1] and *Resource Management in Health and Social Care.*[2] Here are the main factors.

- The use of management principles and practice achieves the most effective level of delegation, having regard to the sustainability of budgets (the size and scope of budgets affect their performance).
- Financial information must be made available to budget managers in time to take remedial action. This implies a low level of reliance upon historical data and the development of reporting systems that provide early warning of problems.

- Reports should be in a format that is easily read and understood. A familiarity with terminology must be fostered. Reports should include a clear statement of financial objectives and should aim for simplicity (difficult when we have access to such a plethora of computerised detail).
- Budget reports must be readily verifiable. Statements must be complete and transparent reconciliations of facts with figures, with variations at each stage identified. The mechanism must clearly connect income with expenditure.
- The system must be compatible with the relevant spending cycle, that is the financial year and the mechanism should make use of the control points characterised by the various events in the supply chain.
- Budget and financial managers must work together to achieve compliance with a mutually agreed financial plan.
- But as part of the delegation process and with the aim of improving performance, budget managers must have clear accountability, as well as authority, for financial management.
- Use must be made of effective intervention techniques and tactics that target significant variations.

Basics of financial management

There have been numerous attempts to define the terms 'management' and 'manager'. Most readers will be familiar with the notions of 'getting things done through people' and the concepts inherent in the principles of delegation. Despite strenuous efforts, they are terms that remain illusive in precision, flexible in interpretation; their characteristic lack of the absolute defies exactitude.

> Delegation is not abdication – but you cannot co-ordinate that which you indifferently control.

For every theory there is a set of limitations that inhibit its full implementation. As opinions change, new ideas find favour and take hold; aspects of this phenomenon can be perceived in the restructuring of health and social care. There are, however, a few general points that can be outlined because they are appropriate to any management situation. Management as an organised activity can be said to embrace the following components.

- **Planning** Every aspect of rational management activity must be subject to a realistic plan even if it is as simple as a diary entry. That plan must be flexible enough to take account of contingencies, but firm enough to be amenable to influence and control.
- **Control** Where there is a plan, its implementation and peripheral activity must be subject to control. Where there is a requirement for

sharing in a cooperative effort or delegation of elements to lower levels in the organisation, the control mechanism implies the acceptability and comprehension of the plan by peer and subordinate groups.

- **Motivation** In organised activity there has to be a significant incentive element. This is a major area of interest to behavioural scientists and has been a fertile research area, giving rise to new insights into the nature of and relationships between achievement and reward.
- **Leadership** This is complementary to motivation. It is the quality that inspires and generates a following. Although leadership has many aspects and styles, which range from the autocratic to the consensus manager, from the pleasant to the unpleasant, it has the common characteristics of imposing a disciplined approach to tasks, generating effort in others and achieving objectives.

Tips from the front office

- Successful leaders and managers are believed to be able to do what they claim they can and will do. It follows that there is an inherent expectation that they will deliver high-quality services within the budgets allocated.
- But in the budgetary systems context, it is the planning and control mechanisms that either facilitate or hinder the achievement of financial objectives.

It seems unlikely that the implementation of a plan without any form of discipline could succeed. This would be partly due to a lack of coordination and partly to a shortage of valid information on how implementation is progressing. The integration of planning and control into a flexible structure (IMIRC) requires the arrangement of information in such a way as to facilitate:

- Implementation – within agreed timescales and at an agreed rate
- Monitoring – facilitates the measurement of progress and signals variations
- Intervention – at an appropriate time to correct a variable
- Revision – takes into account the unexpected
- Control – of the overall process.

Figure 7.1 shows this sequence of events, as described both in *Managing in Health and Social Care* and in *Resource Management in Health and Social Care*.

However, as pieces of data are added to the model two constraints are also introduced. The first is concerned with the timing of reporting and general communication. It is important that reports are both relevant and up to date. The more elements that are added, the more likely it is that delays may occur. The second constraint concerns the possible impairment that might be caused to accuracy where the time factor was considered paramount.

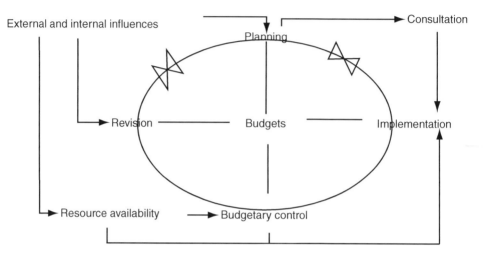

Figure 7.1 Planning and control.

Implications of delay and inaccuracy in financial information

Prior to the development of budgetary management techniques, managers had to rely on historical financial data, which was often months out of date. This was especially true for large and complex organisations where manual adjustments for changes in the levels of assets and liabilities, such as stocks, debtors and creditors, and for payments already made were unbelievably time consuming. In collating this information, the introduction of delays was both common and inevitable. Although the financial information was mostly accurate, the lack of timousness in meeting agreed deadlines and the difficulties in attributing budgets and costs to lower levels of management greatly diminished the capacity to bring significant variations under control.

Nowadays, with computer modelling and budgetary management techniques at a sophisticated level, budgetary information and forecasting are readily accessible. Yet for a number of reasons managers hesitate to take remedial action. With a rapidly expiring time limit, a problem occurs between the desire to conform and the obvious increasing need for expediency. However, corrective action is often frustrated by administrative machinery intended to discourage potentially wasteful endeavours and therefore expediency would never be viewed as an efficient device.

Variations in budget performance must be kept constantly under review so that significant patterns that are likely to escalate are identified at as early a stage as possible. Tendencies to under- or overspend can be indicators. From this, appropriate tactical intervention can be determined and the right action can be made to comply with timescales.

A simplified example based on an arithmetic progession is illustrated in Figure 7.2. It can be seen that when the tendency to overspend is first noted at point t_1, the rate of overspending is $v_1 \div t_1$. If no action is taken by the time the budget period (total time (T)) has elapsed, this overspending will escalate to V. Clearly, the most desirable position is when appropriate intervention is initiated as near to the point where the over- or underspending begins, that is where $t_1 \to 0$.

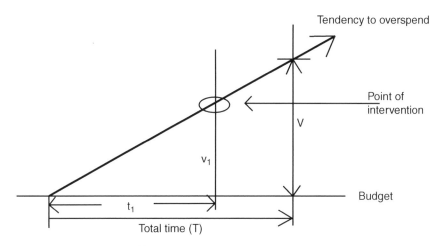

Figure 7.2 Delay and effective intervention.

Delays sometimes occur because of computer failure or where the finance department notices an irregularity that has to be corrected. More often, it is the budget manager who is recalcitrant. Reasons for this inactivity vary from disbelief through to denial. However, the most time-consuming aspect of delay is where a challenge to the veracity of the statement occurs.

The span of management

Business organisations are usually divided into component parts so that a concentration of skilled effort can contribute to more beneficial outcomes. Most readers will be familiar with the concept of the production line in industry and perhaps will have heard of unfavourable comparisons with health and social care organisations. However the basic concepts inherent in specialisation and economies of scale underpin most cooperative effort.

In order to get the maximum benefit from scarce specialised talents and other expensive resources, workloads tend to be concentrated into groupings, the largest being hospitals and the smallest, community teams. This conforms with the business management aim to concentrate on discrete areas of activity. The rationale for the split into specialised divisions can be analysed according to the nature of the split: by profession, function and location.

The dimension that can be embraced within an organisational framework best follows the principles upon which the organisation was originally constructed. This has the advantage of using data that are common to all systems in such a way as to report the same overall position in different ways. It is achieved through according entity status to each part, identifying the range of attributes that can readily be described and which will satisfactorily cover all structural options.

In order to delegate financial management to lower levels of management, it is first necessary to identify the nature of a resource so that it is possible to attribute it to a recognisable department. Broadly, an attribute describes:

- the identity of the resource, for example, a social worker, doctor, piece of equipment
- where the entity is located, for example, in the community, within a hospital ward, in an operating theatre
- what task the resource performs, for example, services to the elderly, clinical services, general surgery
- its relationship to other similar items, for example, the department or budget to which the resource belongs.

If there were no rules to limit the connection between one entity and another, then every entity and its attributes would be treated in the same way. In other words, there would be no discernible structure. However, it is clear that organisational connections are both limited and enhanced by structure. The evolving organisational complexity significantly affects the structure because, as rules are developed, it is clear that other connections can be made, which go beyond the attributes already developed.

The degree and complexity of control can vary. An organisation's degree of sophistication in applying control factors will dictate its place on the spectrum. The main factors to be considered are whether the system is limited to:

- singular financial control
- financial control linked to specific resource purchasing power
- control, purchasing power and output measures linked in complexity
- outcome measures introduced to create composite data
- additional factors.

And the cumulative effect of these definitions is to gather expenditure together so that the big and small spending departments can be readily identified and decisions made as to where budget centres can be placed.

Number of staff

There have been a great number of theories concerned with the numbers of junior staff a manager can reasonably be expected to control. Some have favoured smaller numbers (four to eight) at upper levels, relaxing this rule for lower levels of the organisational pyramid where there is greater specialisation. In the USA, it appears that the most common number in the upper reaches averages out around nine. Recently theorists have tended to take the view that there are too many management variables to be definitive. The resulting principle of the 'span of management' states that there is a limit to the number of subordinates a manager can effectively supervise, but the exact number will depend upon the impact of underlying factors.

Number of departments

If departments are too large, they are difficult to control; if they are too small, then there may be a waste of resources and a likelihood that there is not enough work to maintain a viable specialised team. Although organisations are seldom homogeneous in nature, it is possible to simplify the situation and to calculate how a structure might evolve.

If the total value of the business within an organisation is T, this has to be equal to the total number of departments (n) multiplied by the size of each share (t):

$$T = nt$$

We can apply this simplified equation to a practical example: an organisation that has an annual revenue expenditure of £50m per year. This would be the approximate annual expenditure of a district general hospital trust or a medium-sized community trust. Figure 7.3 demonstrates how the relationship between size of departmental budget and number of departments can be developed. The equation can be refined subsequently to take account of particular circumstances. It is important, however, to grasp the significance of the relationship so that later upper and lower limits can be set.

Levels of management

Depending on the span of management chosen, there will be a relationship between it and the number of levels. Wider spans of management will have flatter organisational structures. Conversely, shorter spans will tend to have more management levels. This is illustrated in Figures 7.4 and 7.5.

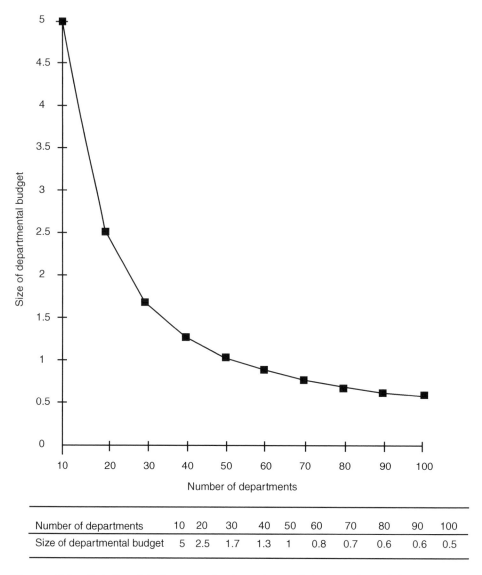

Number of departments	10	20	30	40	50	60	70	80	90	100
Size of departmental budget	5	2.5	1.7	1.3	1	0.8	0.7	0.6	0.6	0.5

Figure 7.3 Relationship between budget size and the number of departments.

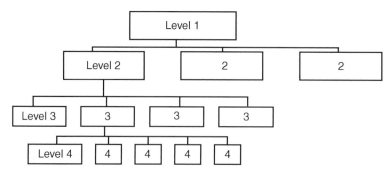

Figure 7.4 Short spans of management: more levels.

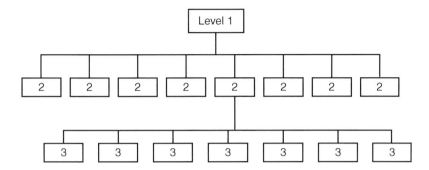

Figure 7.5   Wider spans of management: flatter structure.

The potential for improvement to the environment through adequate financial structures must be balanced with available resources. This is generally facilitated and complemented by developments in both systems and management. However, it is vitally important that the equations that govern the connection between these complex factors are applied in all cases. These may be simplified to embrace the generalities outlined so far:

$$Pa < C$$

$$Pl > C$$

$$Ar > C$$

where Pa is the potential gain to either environment, Pl is the potential loss, Ar is the available resources and C is the cost.

Both types of structure tend to be employed in health and social care. There are frequent wide spans of management to accommodate the diversity of service provision and there are also deep structures with many levels to provide for the intensely specialised nature of some procedures. In such complex organisations there is great potential for wastage resulting from undue overlap or duplication in attributes. Evaluation of structure in the context of business planning seeks to identify such areas. Figure 7.6 illustrates the simplified process.

However, the method of management control is itself another and more subtle factor. With the model in its most simple form, reports may flow with almost complete freedom without any perceivable limitation. The implications of such an arrangement would be far reaching for an organisation because it would pose a challenge for the professionalism that is inherent in these disciplines. It might also mean that the economies of scale that are obtained from managing these functions at a higher level are diminished.

The cost of supporting a structure is a significant factor when considering the capacity for change. Sometimes it is difficult to arrive at the amount of money spent on management. This problem arises mainly because of the

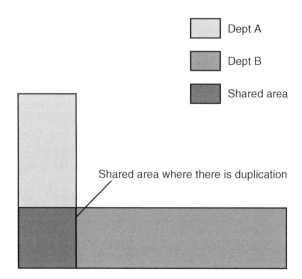

Dept A

Dept B

Shared area

Shared area where there is duplication

Figure 7.6   Departmental duplication.

way accounting methods are applied. For example, there is a dilemma in apportioning the cost of administrative staff dedicated to other professional purposes like social care teams, ward and nursing support groups, medical records, etc. In health and social care management costs can be as high as 6% of the total revenue expenditure and this is an important consideration when any change is contemplated.

It can be seen therefore that as the total cost of service provision grows, the percentage of that cost attributed to management or structure seems to fall. In these terms the best performers are the hospital groups, but the figures do not take any account of the nature of service provision in a community where work is not so concentrated in the one place. In order to compensate for some of these problems, it seems likely that the number of primary care trusts could be halved to a figure somewhere in the region of 150. There are also proposals to reduce the number of strategic health authorities from 28 to 10 in order to address the problem that is external to the provision of services.

Tips from the front office

Make delegation work by adjusting the balance of rules that either limit its scope or liberate creative elements in more junior staff.

• Make a careful definition of the areas and tasks for which the member of staff is responsible.
• Ensure that the person to whom responsibility has been delegated has the complementary authority to carry out the delegated tasks.

- Eliminate any repetitive or time-consuming meetings for clarification or other deferential traits.
- Create a properly accountable environment in which junior staff are given defined powers and authorities, but are also called to account for their progress and activities at intervals.
- Too much interference and you might as well do the job yourself; too little interest in your staffs' activities and coordination will be impossible.

Commonly shared areas

Apart from the departmental overlap that is necessary to vertical and lateral structures, the best known areas where sharing occurs are probably in the provision of administrative support such as ward clerks, receptionists and sub-office staff to individual departments. Another example would be where similar departments exist on the one site. All organisational structures and departments need to be examined to decide whether there is an opportunity for rationalisation of this kind.

Tips from the front office

- Create structures that are flexible and best suit the needs of the organisation.
- Initiate or approve management developments that best suit the needs of the individuals in the organisation.

Key points summary

- Successful budget management must be based on sound organisational compatibility.
- There is a need to resolve conflicts through the establishment of acceptability criteria.
- Project management is the recommended mode for the management of the fixed budgets that reflect minor and major projects and the application of appropriate techniques and methodologies involved in budget management.
- Determination of compatibility and conformance flows from project management and this also provides an indicator of the degree of structural suitability.

- Review and audit of management organisation and structure must take account of:
  - departmentalisation in terms of size and number
  - the shape of structure that is most adapted to organisational needs and not to the availability of managers to fill the gaps
  - the span of management, in terms of narrow or wide spans, numbers and levels must best suit the work to be done.
- Budget structures must conform to the organisational structure.
- Definitive budget structures are necessary to help managers cope with the prevalent business culture.

References

1 Bryans W. *Managing in Health and Social Care: essential checklists for frontline staff.* Oxford: Radcliffe Publishing; 2004. Chapter 7.
2 Bryans W. *Resource Management in Health and Social Care: essential checklists.* Oxford: Radcliffe Publishing; 2005. Chapter 7.

Chapter 8

Tactical intervention

The issues

- Budget reports seldom indicate that expenditure has perfectly mirrored the budget or that there are sufficient funds to meet the forecast.
- Unfortunately, budgets have a depressing tendency to be overspent.
- This reflects the reality that there is never enough money to cover all the demands.
- And, taken together, these are aspects that may be detrimental to a budget manager's development plans.
- However, when budgets are consistently underspent, managers become rightly concerned because they have not been able to buy the human and physical resources they require to maintain standards of care.
- In the longer term, this can damage service viability.
- Underspendings may also signal a need to reallocate financial resources away from a particular service and towards those areas that are overspent.
- Clearly, any suggestion that such a transfer of funds rewards profligate spending is counterproductive.
- Provided it can be justified, a modestly overspent position might therefore be thought to be a budget manager's surreptitious objective.
- If the latter were a prevalent consideration, then a forecasted over-spending could be seen as a self-fulfilling prophesy.
- In order to bring the situation under control, it is therefore important first to tackle any confusion.

Introduction

All resources, including money, are scarce and through the budget management process, the balance between resource and money availability will cause natural variations in spending, which in turn will enable managers to maintain control of their budget position. As a simple example, a tendency to overspend may be reversed by a sudden shortage of a particular resource, thus causing the spending to decrease. Where there are no sudden shortages, budget managers often become adept at creating such situations, such as a short moratorium on overtime.

Whilst juggling these uncertainties, managers will be actively promoting their department and wishing to develop aspects of their service. Such developments may be dependent on:

- new monies specifically provided for service development and improvement; the government claims that new monies have helped the service develop from a budget of £34bn in 1997 to £92bn in 2007 (although, of course, some of this will have been absorbed by inflationary pressures!)

- the expense of another feature becoming redundant or its significance being diminished, for example, in child care, there has been a reduction in the number of children's residential places in favour of family placements
- a service being deemed suitable for provision at a lower level of dependency, for example, the treatment of certain asthma cases by GPs rather than by admission to hospital.

In the latter example, a significant reduction in cases will result in a lower level of hospital income with commensurate consequences for budgets. If this was an unplanned event, then with less money available, there would have to be a reduction in staffing and other resources. Thus it makes sense to anticipate such incidents, such as the consequences of the new GP contract, and have other developments in the pipeline to bring on when resources begin to become free because of the reduced workload.

Consequently, budget setting and profiling inevitably reflect the situation where demand exceeds supply. In a climate of change, however, budget amounts can be subject to dramatic fluctuations according to the cycles of development and reduction that are part of the overall improvement continuum. However, it is imperative that budget managers seek out the reasons for even the smallest ripple so that they can be satisfied with subsequent remedial action.

As we have seen, the causes of budget management problems can be grouped under a variety of different headings:

- incorrect data, for example, items such as an allowance for overtime not being included or a budget incorrectly profiled to take account of seasonal fluctuations
- rate of resource consumption being too high when workloads are falling (and sometimes when they are rising)
- external factors, including resource supply and budget reductions
- underfunding (*see* Chapter 1)
- waste and fraud; when there is no reasonable explanation for a budget to become progressively overspent managers must consider whether it is an indication of possible theft (*see* Chapter 2).

Budget variations

As with the household bills, there is absolutely no doubt that where no attempt is made at control, spending will continue to escalate and we can all testify to the fact that it is doubtful this tendency will be to our advantage. In the case of a large organisation, a similar situation prevails except that underspendings do sometime occur, usually because of resource shortages.

Apparently random variations about the budget target must be brought under control so that over time tendencies to overspend are balanced with tendencies to underspend. This is illustrated in Figure 8.1.

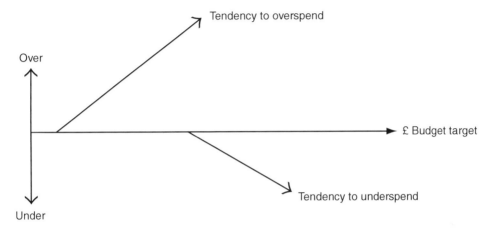

Figure 8.1   Simplified budget variations.

Figure 8.2 illustrates the ideal situation where overspendings are cancelled by later underspendings (shaded areas) to produce a sine-wave type of effect. However, it must be noted that a snapshot at any point in the budget management process will produce an uncharacteristic result. It is important therefore to view the situation in total before any assessment of performance can be made.

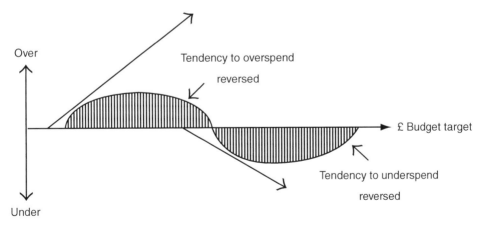

Figure 8.2   Controlling variations.

In Figure 8.3 imaginary points where corrective action may be taken are indicated.

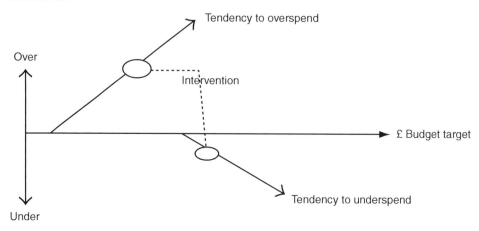

Figure 8.3 Points of intervention.

Against this background budget managers have to bring the situation under control (whether it is an over- or underspending) or at least have initiatives in place that will serve this purpose before they can properly plan improvements. These interlinked functions can be divided into three separate approaches:

- tactical intervention
- strategic initiatives to maintain direction
- planning and developing services.

The links between these three aspects are shown in Table 8.1.

Table 8.1 Links between cause and action

Action →	Tactical	Strategic	Planning
Cause ↓			
Data reliability	X		X
Consumption	X		
External		X	X
Underfunding		X	X
Waste	X		

Successful budget managers have the ability to use the correct level and type of intervention in order to correct any significant deviation. Interventions are of two types: tactical and strategic. Tactics are used on a daily basis but must be applied within the overall strategy of the organisation. For example, managers are usually not permitted to reduce output where it was explicitly intended to expand in a particular area. Strategic intervention, like rationalisation, for example, takes longer to activate and will be reserved for longer-term gains.

Case study

The drug budget for the Near Home Facility was overspent, but by utilising staff expertise, Valerian Grizzle implemented a rigorous rehabilitation regime which was staff intensive. Over an 18-week period, she managed to reduce drug usage and brought the budget back into line. The results are shown in Figure 8.4.

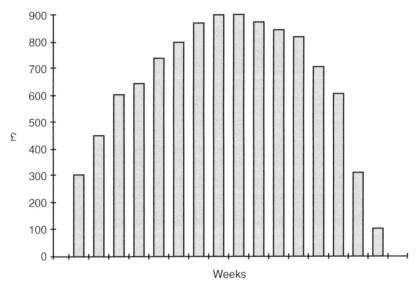

Figure 8.4   Controlling a cumulative drug overspending profile over 18 weeks.

Tips from the front office

- Excessive workloads, whether or not they are being managed within financial limits, are latent hazards that cannot be ignored.
- Another reason for overspendings may be unreliable data. Management must make every effort to ensure that budget information is both correct and verifiable. And, conversely, budget managers have to become adept at identifying and rectifying inaccuracies.
- Defective management arrangements where budgets are not viable, where there is undue dependence upon controlling rather than managing a budget or where expectations are unrealistic can all be contributory factors.
- Intractable problems such as those arising from historical underfunding (inflation, for instance) have to be given due consideration.

- Poor financial competence must also be a concern that must be addressed, for example, through management development programmes; however, it is an internal matter and should not take the burden of blame when reasons for overspendings are complex.

Common forms of tactical intervention

Do nothing

Even in the face of a variation, this option may be the right one for budget management, especially where the variation reported does not conform to previous patterns or is otherwise unexpected. In these circumstances, wait at least until the system has been checked for mistakes.

However, in a climate of change, many managers aim to keep spending below the budget line to provide themselves with a contingency that can be used as the time period progresses and other unexpected priorities emerge. They will therefore be enforcing strict control and taking steps to force spending down. For them, doing nothing is not an option.

Correct any mistakes

As we have seen, mistakes can occur in both the budget calculation (the profiles and additions are incorrect) and the actual amount spent (wrong amounts are charged from other budgets).

Waste

This is a resource manager's ongoing obligation, but any drive on waste can be enhanced by using process quality, as extensively illustrated in *Managing in Health and Social Care.*[1]

Delay

The options for delay in the purchasing/commissioning of new or replacement resources have to be considered in the context of overall performance. It is important to note that although significant savings can be made from the postponement of scheduled works and other schemes, such as painting a ward or departmental block, indefinite delay will inevitably mean that health, safety, weather proofing and general appearance will suffer to the extent that the estate will eventually not be viable (*see* the case study at the end of this chapter).

The expiring time limit is also an important consideration, as fully discussed in *Resource Management in Health and Social Care.*[2] Figure 8.5 illustrates the main points to bear in mind.

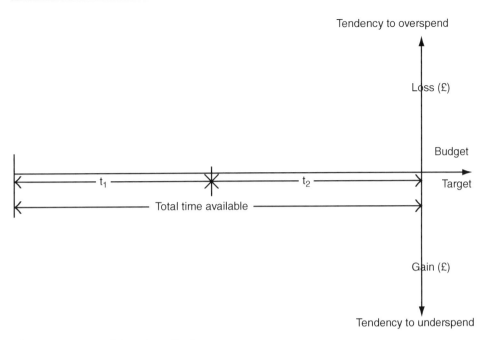

Figure 8.5 Expiring time limit.

In the limited timescale of one stage in the project, variations at t_1 are at risk of being interpreted by a project board keen to manage resources in the best possible way as a financial gain or loss.

- The most desirable circumstances would therefore be when t_1 is near the start-up time.
- The limit of a capacity for tactical intervention happens when t_2 tends to zero. In others words, little or no time remains when the budget manager is made aware of the situation. Project managers must ensure that these indicators are not taken out of context:
  — financial gain (underspending) = potential project failure
  — financial loss (overspending) = poor planning and the project requires urgent revision.

Treatment of both types of variation depend upon the speed at which resources can either be made available in the case of a delay or be mobilised where the budget has been compressed.

Workloads

In contractual situations, managers may decide to reduce workloads to contract levels. This is particularly noticeable in all the public services where, without any commensurate increases, managers may be expected as a duty of care to do more with less.[3] Figure 8.6 illustrates this situation.

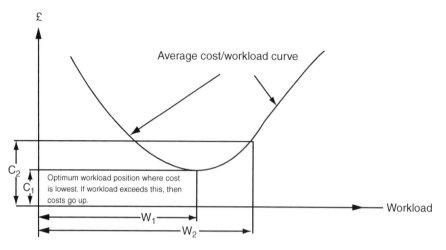

Figure 8.6 More quality activity for less money (Qualm).

In accordance with agreed quality standards, as workload increases, the average cost falls until an optimum point is reached. This is where the most efficient relationship occurs and where the most appropriate budget ($W_1 \times C_1$) should be set. If workload exceeds this agreed limit, to say W_2, the average cost will rise to C_2. And expenditure will be $W_2 \times C_2$. This will result in an overspending of $(W_2 \times C_2) - (W_1 \times C_1)$.

In contrast, it might be more efficient in appropriate circumstances to increase workloads where, for example, an increase may cause the average cost to fall. Generally speaking, though, in situations where workloads have fallen to near zero, the overall future will be reflected in reduced budgets.

Reduce standards

One of the methods used in calculating a budget is to cost the standards that have been set in connection with the quality of patient/client care (*see* Workloads above).[4]

If we take one of these standards and amend the required goals, this will have an effect on spending, such as reversing target attainment initiatives. But it is important to ensure that clients/patients are discharged to the level of dependency appropriate to them (*see* Figure 8.7).

Moratoriums

Sometimes it is appropriate to call a temporary halt to staff recruitment or other commitments such as overtime. This gives time and space to a resource manager wishing to review their operation. A manager may also decide to reduce staffing or other resource levels in other circumstances, for example, when efficiency can be increased using mechanical means. However, where there are pressing contractual obligations, resource levels will have already been defined and a moratorium is therefore not an option.

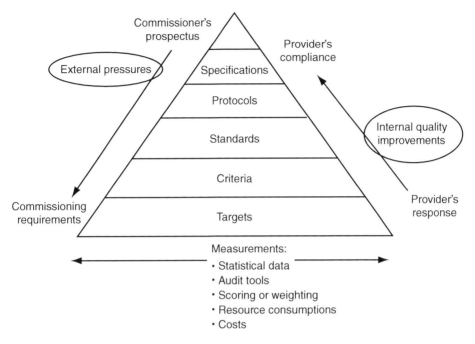

Figure 8.7 Quality regulators.

In all cases, and especially where staffing is the issue, it is imperative that managers observe established protocols for consultation and negotiation with all interested parties.[5] All too often a good idea founders because the agreed format for consultation was not observed and possibly the media carried a premature report that prejudiced progress. It is essential, therefore, that managers become familiar with the established processes within their own organisations. Figure 8.8 shows the main elements of a possible process.

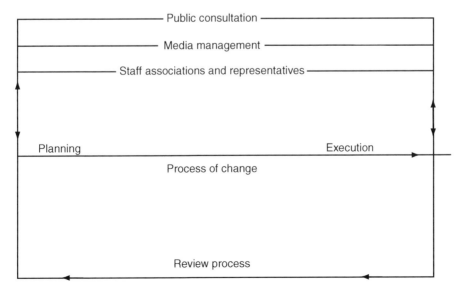

Figure 8.8 Outline consultative process.

Case study

- Bigtown Hospital Trust inherited from its predecessor a facility for the care of the elderly that comprised eight Nissen huts (once part of a World War II military hospital), arranged in opposite pairs and connected by a central corridor.
- The decaying structure was maintained by the estates manager, who appeared to have an endless supply of curved corrugated metal pieces rescued from other similar wartime facilities, so there never seemed to be a need to replace the building. It had its own sewage beds which were still performing their function satisfactorily, so why make changes?
- One of the huts housed the staff dining room and kitchens where rumour had it that cuisine of the highest calibre was available at subsidised rates and that occasionally a small local contract (like a wedding reception for a member of staff) was undertaken at very competitive rates. The staff regarded the facility as a perk of the job.
- Even though the average cost of catering per person was unusually high, several audits revealed no impropriety and were always satisfied with the explanation that there were special dietary needs to cater for. Although the catering budget was always overspent, no action was taken to investigate because the amounts involved were small relatively; so the overspend accumulated.
- Unfortunately, for some obscure reason, staff had to pass through the kitchen area to access the dining room. An inspection revealed that this arrangement was contrary to health and safety regulations, resulting in the kitchen being closed down and all meals being provided from the central kitchen. Although staff were discontented, the change had the gratifying side effect of making considerable savings for the trust.
- The implications triggered a wider study of the facility, including the relative dependency of residents. It was found that the fencing around the filter beds dated back to wartime and no longer provided reliable security to protect elderly residents from accidents. Also the supply of corrugated metal had dried up with the retirement of the estates manager.
- As many of the residents were deemed fit for discharge to the community, and considering the state of the structure, it was decided to close the facility. This resulted in considerable savings, not including the later sale of the woodland to developers.

Key point summary

- The application of tactical interventions are to a degree short-term measures intended to gain time.
- However, they are also important tools that the budget manager becomes skilled in using to keep expenditure within budget limits.

- However, longer-term solutions have to be found in strategic analysis, especially where there are consistent deviations from the agreed budget.
- Before making changes, ensure that all the data contained in the budget are correct.
- Any variation that can be attributed to a historical legacy such as underfunding should be highlighted.
- Examine carefully any unusual or unexplained increases in spending: always bear in mind the possibility of an irregularity arising from a weakness in the system.
- When applying tactical intervention budget managers need to be sensitive to the effects on the quality of patient/client care and to the need for proper consultation.

References

1 Bryans W. *Managing in Health and Social Care; essential checklists for frontline staff.* Oxford: Radcliffe Publishing; 2004.
2 Bryans W. *Resource Management in Health and Social Care; essential checklists.* Oxford: Radcliffe Publishing; 2005. Chapters 5 and 6.
3 *Ibid.* Chapter 8.
4 *Ibid.* Chapter 7.
5 *Ibid.* Chapter 8.

Chapter 9

Prioritising and planning strategic intervention

The issues

- Strategic priorities such as waiting list targets and increasing medical and nursing staff appear to be set at the highest levels.
- And if the number of targets to be attained continues to escalate, then they will certainly diminish local management flexibility.
- Whether there is a deliberate policy of the top-down management characteristic of the desire to gain a tight central control is debatable.
- Certainly in such a large organisation, where there is already such scope for error and misunderstanding, it seems hardly possible that this would be a serious consideration.
- But as things stand, like most initiatives, the advent of planning priorities has its roots in the local scene where various problems have been flagged up initially.
- In this respect, budget and resource managers need to be aware not only of the need to prioritise[1] resources and other demands, but also of their latent capacity to influence the direction[2] the service is going to take.
- However at the same time, unless there are to be significant savings in the longer term, a budget manager's choice of priorities must conform with the organisation's overall strategy so that any bid for additional resources has the best chance of success.

Introduction

It has always been a popular blame-shifting device to hold managers culpable for their apparent inability to prioritise. But what is prioritising? Do we mean according a privileged position to those tasks and demands that have somehow become our favourite and we think will give us maximum profile? And do we make sure that we delegate the multitude of more mundane, time-consuming, odious, or otherwise intricate details to our juniors? In a constant climate of resource scarcity and increasing demand and expectation, we need to be clear about how priorities are graded so that we can stand by our decisions. Problems with accessing, allocating and reallocating resources must be solved rationally.

Sometimes, as well as bidding for additional resources, it is necessary to apply a more powerful strategy, such as contracting out, service rationalisation or stopping a service altogether, which will have more chance of success where tactical intervention is considered or has been ineffective in controlling overspending. These proposals must also be factored into a budget plan, which in turn must fit within the overall strategy.

Within the specific constraints of time, money and structure we must have plans and contingencies to cover any emergencies. In these circumstances, our priorities may have to change according to the feasibility of achieving a particular objective on time. Managers must have a flexible budget planning system through which they can filter demands for additional resources.

Budget planning includes a number of important facets which bind those competing areas together into a cohesive entity. Here is an outline of the process:

- valuing existing resources and assessing their lifespan and potential workload in order to identify any deficiencies[3]
- prioritising competing demands
- assessing organisational capacity to best fit future requirements
- demonstrating capability to build upon specialist facilities, skills and features
- establishing a clear sense of direction or mission
- determining appropriate strategic interventions to create greater efficiency and effectiveness
- ensuring the continued organisational success through willingness to change.

Valuing and prioritising competing demands

Budgeting, rationing and prioritisation are always emotive subjects. Too often there is little or no satisfying feeling of fair play when a decision has been taken. In recognising that there are no easy answers, it is important that managers have a methodology that provides a structure for their consideration. Some of the criteria seem obvious:

- the project must be compatible with the strategic objectives of an organisation to have any chance of success
- a proposal that is too vast in terms of time or money is unlikely to succeed in that form
- cost, price and budget availability will always be limiting factors
- bids should be broken into manageable portions
- identifiable financial and other benefits will add to a project's potential
- availability and time limits will be considerations.

Prioritisation of demands should be made to accord with established criteria by giving each demand a notional score. This will allow you to see which are likely to succeed.[4] In general terms, you should follow the pattern below:

- **Financial planning cycle** Where large amounts of money are involved, make sure your bid is submitted so that it conforms with the financial planning cycle.

- **Strategic direction** Ensure that your projects are in harmony with the overall direction that your organisation has chosen.
- **Additional funding** Look out for extra monies becoming available for cherished initiatives.
- **Health and safety issues** These are always of serious concern and bids or demands that improve conditions can attract a better rating.
- **Cost** Depending on the scale of the cost and other competition for scarce funds, this can detrimentally affect success. Think of breaking up the bid into workable component parts or see whether other options instead of a straight purchase are available. (*See* Chapter 6.)
- **Delivery** Can your proposals be delivered within a reasonable timescale? A long lead time or potential delays can be mean unacceptability.

Tips from the front office

Build on your reputation as a prudent and thrifty manager. Try to ensure that your proposal:

- guarantees a measure of both patient/client and financial improvement
- includes an element of self-finance
- if possible offers improvement through a partnership with a suitable organisation, especially in the case of community services.

Make sure deliveries can be achieved within the timescales laid down, usually before the end of the current financial year. If funds are available for one specific purchase, delivery must be accomplished within the allocated time frame.

Budget planning

Broadly speaking, budget planning should follow a series of steps that identify strengths and weaknesses in the context of the clear establishment of aims and objectives.[5] The evolution of competition to deliver core services requires the identification of discrete areas of business activity that are oriented towards the delivery of services.

Figure 9.1 shows a map of the kind of processes that are involved in budget planning, the main purposes of which are to:

- enhance the particular environmental domain within which each of us works (the historical legacy)
- demonstrate our determination to remain in the business of providing high-quality care through business planning
- secure appropriate levels of funding for budgets.

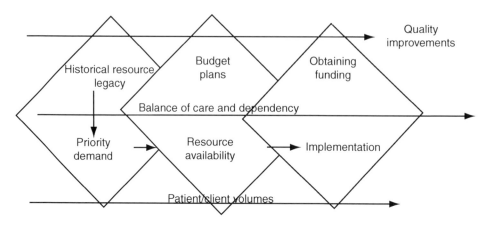

Figure 9.1   Overview of the budget planning process.

The first step in assessing the position is to establish a clear picture of the current position. The process may be broken down into a convenient number of component parts:

- descriptions of current service provisions
- quality initiatives
- analysis of current workloads and dependencies
- resource consumption
- performance levels.

The historical position

It is important to provide a feel for the traditions of service that have so far influenced service development, when it was founded and for what purpose, and any relevant milestone changes that have occurred along the way. The location and accessibility of the service to the catchment, resident, patch or referred population should also be noted. We can follow this with detailed descriptions of current service provision, volume of care and treatments, size of budget, etc. Particular attention should be paid to service elements that are considered to have star quality; for example, keyhole surgery, alternative medicine, respite care, etc.

Quality initiatives

Arising from the historical notes, valued quality of care standards should be noted, together with any initiatives that are being used to accurately measure some of the aspirations. For example, the King's Fund Accreditation packages, quality circles or total quality management should be included where appropriate.

Current workloads and dependencies

These must be assessed, together with current trends, and need in-depth consideration. However, a number of basic statistics are also required:

- population served
- service capacity
- utilisation or take-up.

Resource consumption

The resources needed to support current activity levels have to be produced, verified and analysed. This must include staffing, estate, materials, equipment, funding and systems (SEMEFS).

- **Staffing** A general staffing review indicating deficiencies in key areas, together with imminent retirements, needs to be carried out.
- **Estate** An honest review of the quality and condition of the grounds, buildings and estate services such as water, electricity, gas, telephones, etc., together with priority work being planned, is necessary.
- **Materials** A comprehensive statement must be prepared covering receipt, handling, storage and distribution of materials, goods, drugs, food stuffs, etc.
- **Equipment** An assessment of the condition and replacement plans for all main equipment must be prepared.
- **Funding** Sources and volume of funding need to be analysed together with main expenditure headings.
- **Systems** Systems in use and those planned need to be listed, together with any project management proposals and/or end-stage assessments.

Potential for success and failure

There is little chance of a proposed development succeeding where there is a critical mass of external factors ranged against it. For example, if government policy favours community-based initiatives for certain treatments or care, then there is little chance for a development that is not amenable to that kind of approach. Similarly, if departmental or purchaser preference directs funding towards other schemes, managers whose services are not so favoured must reconsider their options.

However, this does not mean that because external opinion is against a particular proposal, managers must abandon a cherished scheme. Instead they must seek to create an external climate in which their proposals will have a better chance. I will be dealing with this matter in Chapter 10, but for the purposes of this section, we have to accept the realities and work within those parameters.

We want to create a plan that has the best chance of success, one which can readily be translated into the desired action. This means that the relationship between author, executor and environment is sufficiently mature. Generally speaking, capacity to implement a plan can be attributed to the following factors:

- adequate preparation
- sufficient information
- clear objectives
- definitive organisational focus as to internal and external factors
- effective review and monitoring processes
- establishment of control points
- facility for control without undue interference.

Therefore we have to break the process down into manageable parts. The first part is finding out our precise location through careful analysis of the information that is at our disposal.

Benefits

There are a number of benefits that arise from the analysis and management of this information:

- identification of improvements to the internal and/or external environments
- establishment of the significance of limited resources
- need for increased management competence
- demand for more valid information.

Competing factors

The arrangement of competing factors into a workable plan that observes the various limiting factors is generally performed only after considerable consultation. Depending upon the size and scope of the organisation, it emerges as each service aspect and resource element is carefully analysed. Because of its common currency, the central pivot is cost.

Analysis

In this context, SWOT or TOWS analysis should assist. When TOWS is applied, strengths and weaknesses are regarded mainly as internal environmental characteristics; opportunities and threats exist externally. Thus in Figure 9.2 a matrix can be developed which analyses these factors over time.

The initial formulation of the budget plan has to take account of the emerging priorities. It has to comply with the overall process that has been devoted to the realistic consideration of the evaluation:

- external environmental influences
- reality of the internal environment
- performance in care and treatment.

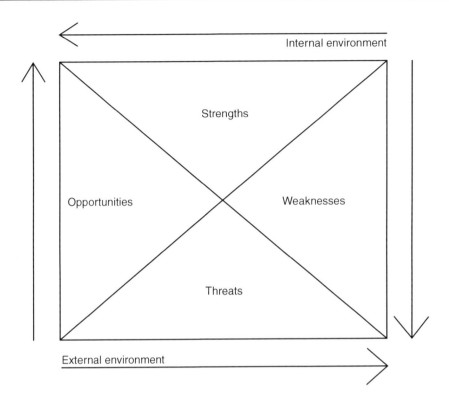

Figure 9.2 Prospective situation using SWOT analysis.

Resource considerations, performance levels and the requirements of the external environment, as represented mainly by the income likely to flow across the boundaries, are reconciled with emphasis on quality and the desired balance of care. This task is undertaken through a combination of financial, statistical and factual analyses.

It is important to build on the perceived positive advantages of strengths and opportunities. Broad ideas can now be prepared to take advantage of prevailing conditions so that the best position is attained in time. The most advantageous position occurs when internal strengths and external opportunities can be maximised.

The source of income or budget that is allocated to any budget holder is representative of the main external influence. Wherever sources are located, income is derived from the provision of service, either as a service provider or as an intermediary in the purchasing chain (whether it is resources or clinical services that are required). In the external scene we find our:

- volumes in terms of patients/clients
- suppliers in terms of physical resources
- sources of income, including statutory funding
- relevant ministerial and government departmental contacts

- statutory regulators and commentators, including the audit commission, arms-length inspection units, etc.
- patient and client support groups, including the individual benefactor
- collegiate support, including staff and professional associations
- coterminous commissioners and providers, including the voluntary sector
- other influential factors, including local authority membership, MPs, the media, etc.

Strategic interventions

As well as tactical intervention, where budget problems remain intractable or where it is thought that better value for money can be obtained, budget managers need to maintain and review their capability to intervene at a strategic level in order to sustain their reputation as economic providers.

Some interventions such as influencing the supply chain[6] are continuing commitments. From initiatives like this will flow improved performance in the domain of purchasing and commissioning, and this will in turn produce longer-term savings. The main interventions in this category follow.

Contracting out

In the hospital service, the contracting out of services by means of competitive tendering has not progressed much beyond domestic and allied services, which account for around 15% of the total budget. By comparison, some other countries have many of their purchased services, including some clinical services, managed in this way. However, it is a cumbersome process that is rewarded only where the amounts of money involved are easily identifiable and are amenable to this type of approach, as in catering services, for example. Figure 9.3 illustrates an outline of the process.

The potential of these initiatives for success depends firstly upon the sensitivity with which the consultative processes are handled, doubtless with many upsets, contradictions and clarifications along the way. The second important consideration is in choosing the most reliable contractor. This can be a protracted and exacting task involving many professional advisers and managers. It is also crucial that a coherent and comprehensive review process is developed and implemented. This must include a capacity for continuous quality assurance and the facility within the terms of the contract for sanctions up to contract termination. Anticipating the development of improvements, for example in catering, there should also be a degree of flexibility in the contract whereby contractors are obliged to maintain pace with new technology.

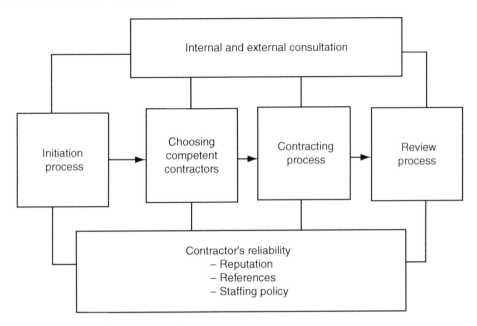

Figure 9.3 Outline contracting out process.

Reducing levels of service

In the strategic sense, service reductions need to follow a carefully chore-ographed consultative process. There are a number of devices which facil-itate these arrangements:

- **Rationalisation** In a climate of change the rationalisation of a par-ticular line or outlet is always a distinct possibility and managers must be prepared for this type of situation.
- **Retract** A retraction of production may sometimes be expedited by developments elsewhere either on the technical/staffing front or with alternative forms of production. This would be a strategic issue and needs to be considered in the broadest possible sense.
- **Close or stop** In extreme cases where budgets have been exhausted, it may be that certain projects can be halted without detriment to the immediate future, for example, painting or routine maintenance programmes.

Partnerships and strategic alliances

A budget manager may enter a strategic alliance or partnership in appro-priate circumstances in order to obtain the best use of resources and to provide a better, more seamless organisational arrangement. However, the potential from the development of partnerships, strategic alignments and collaboration should never be limited to statutory authorities.

Cooperative arrangements with other agencies such as those in the voluntary and charitable sectors at both local and national levels provide access to additional resources and specialist knowledge. As well as this, sometimes it is opportune to develop links with the world of commerce where resource sharing can have beneficial consequences.

In order to achieve these ideals, it is necessary to have workable systems and structures in place so that implementation is facilitated, not hindered by committee. The development of strategic partnerships or alliances implies that there are beneficial consequences for all the partners.

Clearly the creation of formal arrangements to cope with relatively small-scale activities would be counterproductive. On the other hand, where major problems exist, more complex management arrangements may be necessary.

The different types of approach are partnerships, strategic alliances and collaboration.

- Partnerships can be created between two or more people or organisations with either similar types of expertise, for example GPs and solicitors, or different kinds of expertise that together will produce a more effective service.
- Strategic alliances can be similarly created to obtain increased purchasing power. Sometimes in the commercial world, the term describes a situation where a powerful purchaser binds smaller suppliers or service providers into an almost inescapable supply chain.
- Collaboration occurs where there is a willingness to cooperate, but a more formal arrangement is not considered necessary.

The main aspects that must be considered to help determine the level of cooperation needed are outlined below.

- **Definition of specific problem areas** The problem areas need to be coterminous, for example, between health and social care organisations where a seamless service for designated patients/clients can be arranged.
- **Compatible objectives** Joint objectives must conform to the culture and ethos of both prospective partners.
- **Size and scope of the problem** These need to be significant for formal arrangements to be put in place. In other words the process must be worthwhile so that shared resources produce savings that can be spent inwardly, for example reducing duplication of effort.
- **Willing and appropriate partners** There must be a cooperative spirit that motivates joint action and will not generate internal opposition.
- **Expectation of improved outcomes** The arrangement should have clear benefits for clients/patients, for example, the provision of appropriate forms of care at suitable levels.

- **Setting objectives** The arrangement must indicate how objectives are set and how reporting mechanisms that are acceptable are put in place.
- **Implementation process and management** There must be a clearly defined and agreed process for implementation so that all objectives are achieved.
- **Organisation and management development** With the new emphasis on cooperation and revised reporting structures, management development must be made compatible with organisational development. Staff must understand and sign up to the revised arrangements.
- **Evaluation** An agreed system for the evaluation of performance at all levels needs to be in place and, where further changes seem necessary, a system of revision agreed.

It is not possible to have a good or a bad budget plan because flexible business planning must be made an integral part of the overall management process, to be changed and amended as expectation and reality are reconciled. In the implementation stages, the level of performance can therefore be tested provided there are enough definitive material and standards. Necessary improvements can be incorporated as we go along.

Key points summary

Managers have to:

- be competent in their understanding and application of the planning terminology and know exactly how business planning works
- be able to distinguish clearly between their roles as commissioners and providers
- be able to rate tangible and intangible benefits
- define current service levels in terms of background, workloads, dependencies, resources, including finance, etc.
- consider the environmental context and how to evaluate external opportunities and threats against internal strengths and weaknesses
- focus on the boundaries that can be used to match their internal resources against external requirements
- consider the relevance of financial assets and liabilities and their management, and understand their key roles in improving overall performance.

References

1 Bryans W. *Managing in Health and Social Care; essential checklists for frontline staff.* Oxford: Radcliffe Publishing; 2004. Chapter 6.
2 Bryans W. *Resource Management in Health and Social Care; essential checklists.* Oxford: Radcliffe Publishing; 2005. Chapter 8.
3 *Ibid.* Chapter 3.
4 Bryans W. 2004. *Ibid.* Chapter 6.
5 *Ibid.* p. 41–7.
6 *Ibid.* Chapter 5.

Chapter 10

Budget plan implementation

The issues

- Once a budget plan has been agreed its implementation, or something near to it, is mandatory.
- Day-to-day running expenses (revenue expenditure) have a momentum of their own and require management.
- Projects involving change and/or long-term investment need more careful and comprehensive management that often involves more than one budget manager.

Introduction

Ultimate responsibility for the successful implementation of budget plans falls mainly to budget managers. But because of the complexity of health and social care organisations their performance is often dependent on the ability of other managers to obtain the goods and services they require at the right price, time and quality and in the right quantities,[1] or to support them in other coterminous ways.

However, as by far the biggest portion of spending is ongoing and in general terms the day-to-day requirements are known, the management arrangements for procurement and other support mechanisms work pretty well automatically. It is where there is to be a change in emphasis or where there is a large-scale project that problems tend to occur. A change in uniform style might be a simple example of preference or better imagery, but as reorder levels of old stock may be automated, care must be taken to stop ordering the older style and to make sure that existing stocks are used up. Other managers have to be involved.

In the case of large-scale projects where time and money are allocated within specific limits, a more coordinated approach is necessary and this is generally undertaken through project management. This is a technique developed to cope with the intricacies involved in the management of large and complex changes that involve the need for the consensus of a spectrum of professions.[2] For example, it is used extensively in the planning and commissioning of major works and has also been refined to assist the design and implementation of large-scale computer systems.

A variant has also been successfully applied to the budget management process where longer-term investment, such as the management of change, is involved. In order to illustrate these concepts more fully, an example of Bigtown Hospital Trust's simplified budget plan for the current year is used.

Bigtown Hospital Trust's simplified budget plan

Background

Bigtown Hospital Trust, together with a mental health trust, were established following a local restructuring of hospital services and the closure of Smalltown Infirmary. This was accompanied by a renewed determination to work with other providers in the area both to develop a seamless service, especially for vulnerable groups, and where possible to reduce costs through a better balance of care, resource sharing and other initiatives. Accordingly, Bigtown Hospital Trust enjoys a cordial relationship with Bigtown Social Services Department, the mental health trust, the community health care services trust, local GPs, etc. It has also been able to develop a number of mutually beneficial arrangements that have already improved services for the Bigtown population as a whole.

However, the restructuring has also caused a re-evaluation of service provision and a reworking of the budget for the Near Home Facility joint venture.[3,4]

The total amount of combined spending for a 300,000 population is given in Table 10.1 and illustrated in Figure 10.1.

Table 10.1   Estimated combined annual expenditure for health and social care

Service	£m
Family health (GPs, dentists, etc.)	118
Acute hospital care	160
Primary health	12
Maternity and child health	20
Mental health	32
Care of elderly	90
Other	68
Total	500

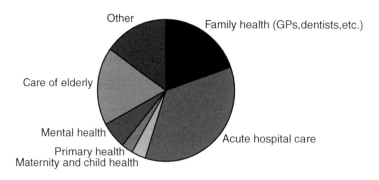

Figure 10.1   Service shares of combined spending.

Service profile

Bigtown Hospital Trust serves a population of approximately 300,000, employs around 4,000 full-time and part-time staff and treated 400,000 patients last year. The headline treatment figures are shown in Table 10.2.

Table 10.2   Headline treatments

A&E	65,000
Out-patients	260,000
Day patients	12,000
In-patients	63,000
Total	400,000
Operations	22,000
Births	3,700

Day patient activity has risen significantly since the day surgery unit opened five years ago. This is shown in Table 10.3 and Figure 10.2.

Table 10.3   Rise in number of day patients over five years

Year	Day patients
Current year	12,000
4	10,000
3	9,000
2	7,000
1	5,000

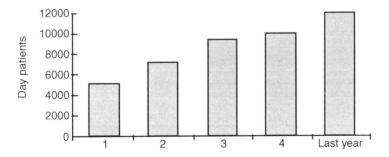

Figure 10.2   Rise in number of day patients over five years.

However, the rise in day patients, together with shorter lengths of stay for in-patients, has not reduced the number of beds being used because of the closure of nearby Smalltown Infirmary. In order to accommodate the extra pressure from the closure of Smalltown Infirmary, beds in St Bedifuls were reallocated as follows:

- 30 beds in the maternity unit, which was half vacant due to a successful policy of early discharge

- 50 beds in surgical specialties, due to the increasing use of minimum invasive techniques
- 50 beds available because of the relocation of the integrated mental health unit to the local mental health trust.

Indeed, the result has been an increase in in-patient activity due to an influx of referrals by the mainly rural population that lives in the Smalltown and Bigtown hinterland.

As with many rural areas, there has been a drift away from agriculture by the younger generations in favour of towns and cities, leaving behind a proportionately older population on the land. One worrying feature of this has been to increase the number of over 80s occupying acute beds (about 42%). This has in turn led to an in-depth review of the Near Home Facility, which is a joint venture with community services, aimed at ensuring that vulnerable patients receive the best and most appropriate care and that those with complex requirements have an appropriate form of care assessed before discharge to the community.

Resources

The budget for the current year is shown in Table 10.4. Debts amount to £8m and the overall budget has been reduced by £4m. Included in non-payroll are budgets for significant items that are causing concern: drugs, medical and surgical equipment, patients' appliances, energy and contracted out-services. The breakdown is shown in Table 10.5.

Table 10.4   Budget outline

Revenue	£m	Totals
Payroll	110	
Non-payroll	50	160
Capital schemes		10
Free funds		8

Table 10.5   Non-payroll budgets causing concern

Details	£m
Drugs	9
Patients' appliances	1
Medical and surgical equipment	9
Energy	1
Contracted-out services	5

- Both drugs and medical and surgical equipment have shown an increase in expenditure of 20%, which is well in excess of inflation. The care of the elderly team were impressed by the results of the rigorous rehabilitation regime in the Near Home Facility, which over an 18-week period reduced drugs usage and brought the budget back into line. A number of separate investigations into general prescribing policy are being conducted and participation in strategic purchasing initiatives is in hand.
- A working party has been set up to evaluate the appropriateness of the transfer inwards of staffing and funds to cover the additional costs involved with Smalltown Infirmary and the transfer outwards of resources to the mental health trust.
- In the light of the fact that energy costs have also risen and are expected to escalate further, energy conservation, together with a number of solar and wind power proposals, are under consideration.
- Spending on patients' appliances has always proved difficult to control and this budget is currently under review. However, strenuous efforts by appliance officers and the physiotherapy department to recover items that are no longer in use are being pursued.
- The contractor for domestic services withdrew from the contract on mutually agreed terms and so the trust has had to take the service back in-house. While consultations continue with trade unions, an interim agreement has been reached so that management can review the situation with a view to testing the market for all or part of the service.

Near Home Facility

The main objectives of the partnership arrangements for the facility were the provision of a seamless service for older and disabled patients/clients and to:

- facilitate the discharge of elderly and vulnerable patients from higher levels of care and their admission to other more appropriate levels
- avoid the need to rush patients/clients into life-changing decisions by giving them time for reflection
- provide more suitable cost-effective alternatives to unnecessarily long stays in hospital
- further reduce the elderly population occupying acute beds
- obtain better discharge rates in this category of patient/client.

A number of options were considered for the siting of the new facility: the original best choice was the Smalltown Infirmary refurbishment, but in the light of developments it was finally decided to locate the facility in the old sanatorium building in the grounds of St Bedifuls. The facility had three important characteristics:

- an assessment and rehabilitation unit with a strict discharge policy

- the limited provision of short-term respite care beds for community carers
- community support through the already established pathways of care teams.

The last stage of the project, the commissioning of the rehabilitation unit, was initiated at the beginning of the current year.

The original budget,[5] together with the amount uncommitted in the previous periods, increased bids received since and the agreed budget for the final stage implementation are shown in Table 10.6.

Table 10.6 Budget for the final commissioning stage

Detail	Original (£k)	Unspent (£k)	Increased bid (£k)	Final (£k)
Capital cost of refurbishment	500	100	150	130
Revenue costs:				
• assessment unit	560	0	0	0
• rehabilitation unit	120	100	120	110
• pathways of care teams	57	0	0	0
• rehabilitation and follow-up	47	0	30	25
• management development	50	20	25	20
Totals	1,334	220	325	285

Although not large scale, the refurbishment of the unit, extra staffing and coordination of other resources are complex in terms of both resource mixes and organisational requirements. With regard to the latter, in order to secure the greatest chance of success, it is most important to ensure that all professional views are properly represented whilst at the same time keeping the structure simple. Otherwise the arrangement will be ineffective. For the final-stage management team this meant including representatives from the four main organisations: social services, community health, GPs and hospital. In addition, representatives from specialist areas such as business departments and PAMs were required for their specific expertise. Project board membership was restricted to the director of social services and the chief executive of the Bigtown Acute Hospital Trust. Project team membership was therefore agreed as follows (not necessarily in order of importance):

- project manager/head of Near Home Facility
- manager of services to the physically handicapped
- manager of home nursing services

- member of community occupational therapy services
- representative from hospital physiotherapy
- senior representative from supplies
- senior representative from personnel
- other co-opted members appropriate to the stage or with special interest, for example, a consultant in physical medicine.

In the light of experience with previous stages, the trust board recognised that within the total project budget of £285k the wide spectrum of resources being purchased for or released into the system would be difficult to control.

Final stage management

Management of commitments

In interim periods where there is uncertainty about deliveries or other resource problems that create potentially erratic behaviour, comparisons with set targets can be difficult to interpret. Expenditure trends are not therefore in themselves amenable to or reflective of untoward changes. Similarly, in project management where large-scale and complex activities have to be coordinated, the effects of management decisions within stages are not always constant or consistent. This results in resources being purchased or released into the system in an apparently haphazard way. Budget or resource targets are not therefore easily divisible in equal segments so that monitoring and possible intervention are facilitated.

Irregular trends and patterns make comparison with targets difficult. The ability to manage within an overall plan calls for a different approach. The movement from a purely historical record-keeping situation and towards a better financially managed environment requires both a more secure information base and a different kind of approach to budget management.

When a spending direction has been established, tasks are divided, budgets planned and profiled and targets for a particular period set. A process must be created that both ensures their achievement and rationally measures progress towards that achievement. This mechanism should be easily amenable so that appropriate timely intervention is facilitated. We want to be able to:

- make comparisons between progress and the project plan
- detect deviations from that project plan
- determine how and when to intervene.

As well as participating in partnerships arising from the commissioning process, the exercise of purchase and distribution of resources and services covers the whole spectrum of spending by supplies and personnel managers. It includes the purchase of staff, equipment, materials and services. These are constantly consumed by the organisation's internal environment. It is the rate of consumption of a particular item or group that is the dominant factor in the overall cost of the service provided.

However, it is a little understood fact that, as a direct result of supply and personnel managers' key strategic position between internal budget managers and the external market place, they significantly influence the level of the budget set and the time limit upon which delivery depends. At the outset, therefore, it is vital that supplies and personnel managers accurately measure the rates of consumption and likely lead times so that they influence the setting of initial financial and time targets beneficially.

In order to gain control of the spending cycle, it is necessary to both clearly identify the purchasing source and keep a record of the various stages through which the commissioning episode will pass. It is also important that budgets are managed in such a way that uncontrolled events, which can result from an inability to plan, are reduced to manageable proportions. This means that not only new projects but assets nearing the end of their useful and cost-effective life are identified in sufficient time to plan for their replacement or redeployment. Through this process the supply manager is placed in a better position from which to judge how best financial resources may be allocated during a particular financial period. The advent of a financial episode can therefore be predicted at a specific time and place, and the budget set accordingly.

Provided that existing resources are subjected to the management process, their need for replacement can generally be signalled through an automated mechanism. This will commence the commissioning cascade, which should terminate with the fulfilment of all the objectives. The progress of the episode must be tracked throughout so that comparison with the budget is possible. Significant deviations must be identified so that intervention in either curbing the spending programme or re-allocating financial resources is facilitated.

Sometimes the combined effect of built-in obsolescence, poor financial foresight and long-term implications of cash ebb and flow threaten the validity of cash-flow planning and may herald an imminent catastrophe. In the microsystem, although working within delegated authority, budget managers may implement a spending activity on expertise or goods and services at infrequent and perhaps unfortunate intervals so that the matching of income and expenditure has a haphazard and at best fortuitous appearance. In these cases, the supplies and personnel managers have to take account of the potential deficit or surplus.

This evolution from passive record-keeping to more active participation, intervention and regulation does not signify a rejection either of historical record or of obligation. Indeed, the implications of past decisions have as important a bearing on current opportunities as have previous experience.

The methodology reconciles sources of origin for management decisions, contracts and other commitments with deliveries/appointments as they are taken up. This provides a much more accurate barometer of performance within financial targets and deadlines.

The management of commitments uses both 'money and time balances remaining' in a budget to help managers determine future actions (*see* Chapter 6). This process is illustrated in Figure 10.3.

- The budget manager receives an allocation of time and money, but clearly account also has to be taken of the agreed plan and the opportunities for management.
- Although these resources should represent a certain level of purchasing power, because of marginal activity, it is unlikely that this strict relationship will be maintained.
- The budget manager must inevitably have regard to this situation and through it attempt effective management.
- At the outset, therefore, it is important that the right time frame and the correct budget are allocated.
- This involves taking up some of the time to assess the exact financial consequences.

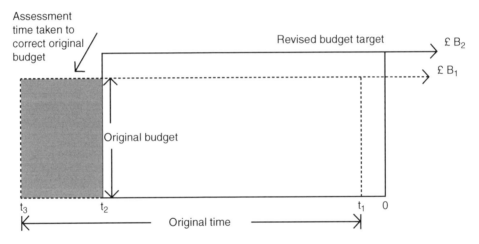

Figure 10.3 Establishing the financial episode.

The limiting situations, as shown in Figure 10.3, are as follows:

- at t_3 the original time span within which the task was to be completed was at its maximum, but the estimated budget B_1 was too low
- at t_2, following fuller research, quotations, etc., a revised higher budget B_2 was allocated, together with an extension of the time limit
- between t_2 and zero (the expiry of the time limit) a firm commitment to purchase or release resources must be made so that the objectives may be met. Also during this time, efforts must be made to ensure that either the two objectives are met or an alternative is found
- at zero there must be a reconciliation between budget and achievement.

Perhaps the most challenging aspect of developing this monitoring feature is the rationalisation of decision packages within the money/time framework. Although these packages will by their very nature exceed resources available in the interim, they must be made to equal expenditure and budget in the final analysis. This is illustrated in Figure 10.4.

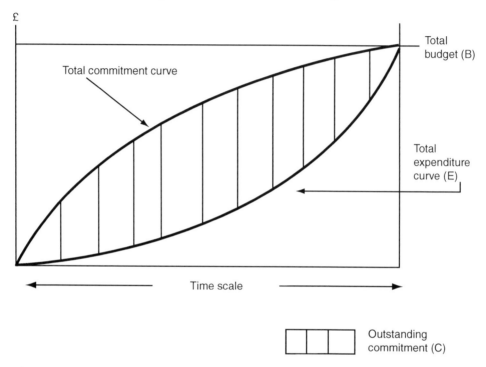

Figure 10.4 The basic commitment and expenditure model, where B is taken to represent the total budget available, E is expenditure or the release of resources and C is the outstanding commitment.

During the project period, commitment to expenditure will be greater than actual expenditure. Indeed, commitment may at times be greater than the budget available, but this is controlled within the time limit through the management process.

In this case study, it was discovered that despite what appeared to be a controlled expenditure trend, partly because of low estimating and partly as a result of an inadequate budget, pipe-line commitments entered by supplies and personnel exceeded the budget by £50k. This is illustrated in Figure 10.5.

Having regard to the time scale, budget management centres are on a constant review of outstanding commitment in the context of current delivery pattern. Towards the end of the period, the position will be modified by extracting commitments which are unlikely to come to fruition in time, and other more promising items will be substituted, the original schemes becoming, where appropriate, a commitment in the new period.

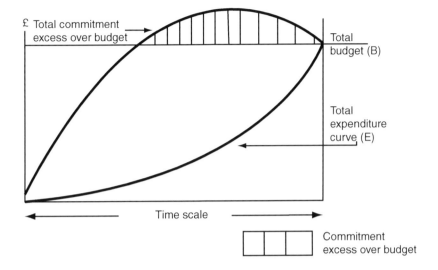

Figure 10.5   Excess commitments.

Conclusion

The budget planning process leads managers through a series of steps that identify strengths and weaknesses in the context of the clear establishment of aims and objectives. The evolution of a competitive market for the delivery of core services requires the identification of discrete areas of business activity that are oriented towards the delivery of services. Figure 9.1 shows a map of the kind of processes that are involved in business planning, the main purposes of which are to:

- enhance the particular environmental domain within which each of us works (the historical legacy)
- demonstrate the determination to remain in the business of providing high-quality care through business planning
- secure appropriate budget contracts.

Key point summary

- Commitment management is an active rather than a passive method of monitoring project budget performance.
- It takes account of current expenditure and any other item that the budget manager has requested.
- The methodology is sophisticated and can be applied to any form of project management.
- Commitment management is based on the theory that the balance remaining in a budget after deducting all those items that will be charged to it during the financial period can be effectively

managed so that spending and budget totals are made to coincide at the end of the period.
- Where, at any time during a financial period, commitments are in danger of exceeding the budget, contracts must be either deferred to a more acceptable time or cancelled or the budget increased.

References

1 Bryans W. *Resource Management in Health and Social Care; essential checklists.* Oxford: Radcliffe Publishing; 2005. Chapter 8.
2 Bryans W. *Managing in Health and Social Care; essential checklists for frontline staff.* Oxford: Radcliffe Publishing; 2004. Chapter 1.
3 *Ibid.* Chapter 1.
4 Bryans W. 2005. *Ibid.* Chapter 6.
5 *Ibid.* p. 97.

Process quality in financial and business management

The efficiency and effectiveness of administrative and financial systems depend heavily upon the competence of all staff; the active participation of all those in clinical or social disciplines is particularly required, even though their main priorities are naturally centred on their patients and clients. Unfortunately, frontline staff do not necessarily have expertise or experience in business matters.

Serious consequences can result from simple mistakes, negligence or ignorance. They can cover a wide spectrum, including complaints, claims for negligence or non-compliance with contractual obligations, budget deficits and diminished performance. Even though they are not life-threatening, such consequences can be measured in terms of both morale and money, reducing the time and money that can be spent on patients/clients. They can therefore have a debilitating effect on the organisation.

It makes sense, therefore, to perform business tasks correctly so that the bureaucracy works smoothly and at a minimum cost. It follows that budget managers at all levels in any organisation can exercise a consider-able element of budget management and control by ensuring that certain protocols and procedures are constantly observed by all their staff.

Consequences of process failure

There are frequent occasions when frontline staff find themselves con-fronted by urgent problems associated with financial, legal or administra-tive matters for the first time and are unsure how to proceed.[1] In these situations, inexperience, negligence, inaccessible advice or ignorance of sound guidance can lead to all sorts of serious problems that include the potential for fraud, ineffectiveness and resource waste. The resulting process failure is illustrated in Figure A1.1.

Process failure results in wasted time and effort in correcting errors and making endless adjustments to take account of an escalating list of mis-takes. It causes frustration, loss of motivation and the opportunity for fraud through what is perceived to be management ineffectiveness. It can also be partially responsible for poor industrial relations.

Whilst every authority and trust has its own rules and regulations, these are often not immediately available to the hard-pressed ward sister, staff nurse, night staff or a multitude of other staff: indeed, it is impossible to keep the thousands of staff on an acute hospital site properly briefed.

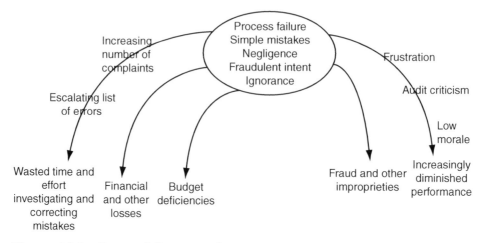

Figure A1.1   Process failure cascade.

However, without contradicting the rules or regulations, resource and budget managers can help to avoid process failure by implementing a systematic business and financial process quality programme that seeks to:

- do the right thing
- at the right time
- every time.

Benefits of implementing process quality

Some of the main components of such a structured programme are listed below and will help to save money:

- reviewing and implementing sensible arrangements for the handling and recording of gifts and cash
- seeking to apply greater influence on supply chain management
- improving and developing finance departmental relationships, for example, ensuring that deadlines set by the paymaster are met
- increasing business, administrative and budget competences through proper training and management development programmes
- positively participating in various processes, such as planning and organising meetings
- assembling coherent cases for additional resources
- helping to improve existing conditions
- building up and maintaining a comprehensive source of reference.

Here is a checklist of the benefits of process quality (Figure A1.2 gives an overview of the expected benefits as action is taken):

- reduced level of physical losses and waste in time, effort and money
- budget savings, reflected in increased resource capacity and the ability to handle more patients/clients

- lower overall costs with commensurate collateral advantages
- improvement in confidence and competence
- enhanced reputation and more secure market connection
- higher levels of patient/client satisfaction and increased capacity to deal with more patients/clients
- reduced sickness, absenteeism and staff turnover.

These benefits can be quantified to give a comparison between the forecast and the reality.

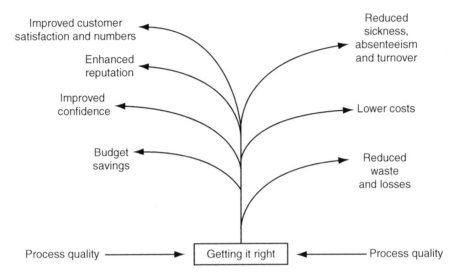

Figure A1.2 Process quality in action.

Reference

1 Bryans W. *Managing in Health and Social Care: essential checklists for frontline staff.* Oxford: Radcliffe Publishing; 2004.

Confidentiality in business dealings

In addition to the absolutes inherent in the management of patient/client information, confidentiality is an important issue in the day-to-day running of health and social care organisations.[1]

Business information

Business information can be extremely valuable intellectual property because it centres on the acquisition of huge quantities of resources and the payment of massive amounts of money. Most business and financial information has to be shared between certain parties, for example, in the case of a job application or a contract tender. Sharing of information is also necessary to complete certain transactions, for example, payroll involves the personnel and the salaries and wages departments. However, if such information falls into the wrong hands, where unfair advantage can be gained, it can cost health and social care organisations dearly.

In order to obtain the best value for money, competition between suppliers for contracts, and between candidates for jobs, is the normal process. Contracting is entirely dependent upon the integrity of the system, which ensures that material facts, figures and prices quoted by one individual are not passed on to a competitor. Such confidentiality also helps to eliminate any potential price fixing between contractors.

Care must also be taken to be clear about the conditions that constitute corruption so that staff who come into contact with suppliers can avoid situations in which they feel to be under an obligation.

Personal information

On a national basis, up-to-date data sets for 1.3m staff covering over 2,000 grades include a wide spectrum of intricate detail. Therefore it makes good economic sense to have integrated systems linking the mechanics of recruitment, continued employment and termination with payroll so that the data can be shared.

However, to be effective, preserve confidentiality and protect the integrity of each department, as well as make accurate payments to the appropriate personnel, the system must have graded levels of divulgence of information. For example, staff in personnel should not be able to act on their own to make payments, which could be for fictitious recipients; on the other hand, payroll staff should not be able to change or generate new pay records without clearance from personnel. Similarly, confidential information such as details of disciplinary matters held in the personnel system or tax details held in the payroll system must not be accessible to inappropriate system users.

In view of the possibility of criminal or even terrorist activity, which could centre around keyholders for example, there must be no external divulgence of basic data such as staff names and addresses from any source, except in certain defined circumstances. However, normal inquiries such as confirmation of a person's income for the purpose of obtaining a mortgage may be released provided that person approves in writing.

Health and social care organisations have a duty of care to protect sensitive information from unauthorised access. Such information may be the details contained in staff records and other personal documents or may be information about suppliers, gathered in the course of the contracting process. For example, staff requesting advice or assistance from management may feel obliged to give intricate background detail that they would otherwise prefer to keep private.

Fundamentally, the confidential nature of personnel/payroll records protects the organisation from abuse and the individual from identity fraud and theft.

Conclusions

Health organisations and their staff have a clear duty of care to protect confidential data and other sensitive information from extraneous interests and influences. Laxness, casual attitudes and general indifference to the importance of confidentiality should be actively discouraged. Staff must also deny access to data and information in all but the most obvious circumstances where, for example, denial would result in a disadvantage to the individual and that individual has given approval in writing.

It follows, therefore, that in order to observe their obligations, organisations need to secure their personnel, supplies and finance systems within their own administrative framework. The following checklist outlines the key issues.

- Ensure that clear instructions on appropriate behaviour for staff and board members when conducting their legitimate business are available.
- A strict code of conduct regarding confidentiality should be in place and the organisation's attitude to the serious nature of any breach should be made clear.
- The same principles should be applied to any person or commercial organisation seeking to gain confidential information.
- Make sure that employment and contracting are regulated so that documents such as applications and tenders are properly received, recorded and kept safe until they are due to be considered.

- Strictly apply closure dates and times so that no late applicants (potentially with prior knowledge) are ever considered.
- Ensure tenders are kept safely by an independent party and opened in accordance with existing protocol, recording the relevant details at that time.

The losses due to a breach in confidentiality can be both tangible (in the sense of having to pay too much for contracted services that were corrupted by undue influence) and intangible (as in diminished staff morale and impoverished reputation).

Reference

1 Bryans W. Minding your own business. *Health Management*. 2006; **September/October**: 22-3.

Selecting competent contractors

The search for competent contractors is an intrinsic part of all purchase/payment systems.[1] However, ignorance of the essential steps or negligence in applying established protocols will inevitably lead to losses and possibly to the collapse of the process. Resources are wasted as a result. For example, lack of consultation seems to have been one of the factors leading to the recent failure of the high-profile contract notice inviting contractors to bid for the management of financial, administrative and human resources.

Where a supplier's acceptability for an engineering, a building or a service contract is subject to protracted analysis and the careful sifting of detail, it saves time to do the preparatory work in advance. Here are some of the key issues.

Feasibility

In cases where a major shift in practice is contemplated, a feasibility study needs to be undertaken. Situations include:

- the method of delivering or commissioning goods or services
- the introduction of new technology or developments
- the purchase of new products
- fresh approaches to care and treatment
- contracting out and out-sourcing
- the rationalisation of clinical and other services.

Stimulating competition and ensuring equality

The system of competition is used in the hope of obtaining the best value for money, which often means that goods and services are not sought primarily on the lowest price rule. The emphasis is always on economic considerations rather than cheapness.

Within the process, it is important to make sure that all potential contractors enjoy an equality of opportunity. In order to ensure equality and where the proposed contract is for an existing service, interested internal management teams must be given reasonable opportunity to submit an in-house tender.

After initial discussions, the size and scope of the proposed contract should be decided so that the request for interested contractors is pitched at the right level, whether that is local, regional, national or international. It is also customary to stipulate all the relevant legislative and regulatory requirements clearly so that there can be no misunderstandings about them.

Ethical and moral issues

Competent contractors are generally expected to conform to any agreed codes of conduct or ethical positions adopted by heath and social care organisations. Here is a quick checklist of the relevant points.

- **Compatible objectives** Prospective contractors need to demonstrate that the nature of their business is not in conflict with the moral or cultural aspirations of the contracting organisation, such as attitudes to smoking, substance abuse and health or green issues.
- **Transparency** Competent contractors should have no interest or influence that is prejudicial to fair dealing or transparent contracting. They should never be in a position where they can sway the course of the tendering or contract process.
- **Local economy** Although it is no longer an obligation, the effects of a particular proposal upon the local economy should always be considered. In addition, the appropriate use of the media for the purposes of maintaining good relations should always be implemented.
- **Staff considerations** In order to avoid any unrest due to rumour, established protocols concerning staff consultation must be strictly observed.
- **Confidential information** The essential duty of care of all organisations to protect confidential information includes business information (*see* Appendix 2).

The process of competition

The process, designed to save time in the longer term, is a protracted one, which requires participants from a variety of disciplines to work together in a form of project management. Here is a list of the relevant conditions.

- **Reputation** Competent contractors must show that they have the capability to adhere in all respects to the physical conditions, such as making a quality product or, in the case of patient/client care, have the ability to provide the quality of services required. Their reputation as a producer or provider of a service has to be acceptable and they must show by means of references to work previously undertaken that their record is satisfactory.
- **Capacity** To be considered, competent contractors have to show that they are a large enough organisation to handle the volumes at the stated price and deliver to the requisite destinations at the times and frequency stipulated.
- **Staffing structure and policy** A competent contractor will be able and delighted to demonstrate that their internal organisation adequately reflects the tasks required and that they operate staffing policies commensurate with those required by health and social care organisations.

- **Qualifications** In complex contracts, particularly in contracting out and in the commissioning of patient/client services, the requisite levels of competence of staff must be demonstrated.
- **Regulation and legislation** Competent contractors must show that they conform in all respects to the regulations that govern the way their organisation performs.
- **Sub-contracting** In large contracts, most health and social care organisations will want to know whether there will be an element of sharing or out-sourcing and, if that is the position, then they may wish to ensure that all the above conditions are fulfilled by the sub-contractor.
- **Audit or other types of inspection** Contractors and health and social care organisations must agree on the methods for ensuring that, if the contract is awarded, there is consistent compliance with all the conditions listed.

Reference

1 Bryans W. Competent contractors. *Health Management.* 2007; **January/February**: 28–9.

Useful websites

- www.doh.gov.uk/finman
- www.doh.gov.uk/waitingtimes
- www.hm-treasury.gov.uk
- www.dpp.org.uk
- www.auditcommission.gov.uk
- www.communitycare.co.uk
- www.integratedcarenetwork.gov.uk
- www.kingsfund.org.uk

Recommended reading

- Baxter C (ed). *Managing Diversity and Inequality in Health Care*. London: Bailliere Tindall/RCN; 2001.
- Bryans W. *Managing in Health and Social Care: essential checklists for front-line staff*. Oxford: Radcliffe Publishing; 2004.
- Bryans W. *Resource Management in Health and Social Care: essential checklists*. Oxford: Radcliffe Publishing; 2005.
- Codling S. *Benchmarking*. Aldershot: Gower; 1998.
- Glasby J. *Hospital Discharge: integrating health and social care*. Oxford: Radcliffe Medical Press; 2003.
- Glasby J and Littlechild R. *The Health and Social Care Divide: the experiences of older people*. Bristol: Policy Press; 2004.
- Ham C. *Management and Competition in the NHS* (2e). Oxford: Radcliffe Medical Press; 1997.
- Hyde J and Cooper F (eds). *Managing the Business of Health Care*. London: Bailliere Tindall/RCN; 2001.
- Leathard A (ed). *Interprofessional Collaboration: from policy to practice in health and social care*. London: Brunner-Routledge; 2003.
- Maxwell R. Quality assessment in health. *BMJ*. 1984; **13**: 31– 4.
- McDonald R. *Using Health Economics in Health Care: rationing rationally?* Buckingham: Open University Press; 2002.
- Moulin M. *Delivering Excellence in Health and Social Care*. Buckingham: Open University Press; 2002.
- Peck E. *Organisational Development in Healthcare: approaches, innovations, achievements*. Oxford: Radcliffe Publishing; 2005.
- Phillips A. *The Business Planning Tool Kit: a workbook for the primary care team*. Oxford: Radcliffe Medical Press; 2002.
- Semple Piggot C. *Business Planning for Health Care Management*. Buckingham: Open University Press; 2000.
- Stewart R. *Evidence-based Management: a practical guide for health professionals*. Oxford: Radcliffe Medical Press; 2001.
- Walshe K. *Regulating Healthcare: a prescription for improvement?* Buckingham: Open University Press; 2003.
- Young A and Cooke M (eds). *Managing and Implementing Decisions in Health Care*. London: Bailliere Tindall/RCN; 2001.

Index